MORBID OBESITY

MORBID OBESITY

WILL YOU ALLOW IT TO KILL YOU?

Eduardo Chapunoff, M.D., F.A.C.P., F.A.C.C.

To order additional copies of this book, contact:
Xlibris Corporation
1-888-795-4274
www.Xlibris.com
Orders@Xlibris.com
61098

CONTENTS

EXCERPTS FROM REVIEWS AND QUOTES ON

ANSWERING YOUR QUESTIONS ABOUT HEART DISEASE AND SEX

Eduardo Chapunoff, M.D.

Foreword by
Arnold A. Lazarus, Ph.D.
Distinguished Professor Emeritus of Psychology
Rutgers University

FINALIST
ForeWord Magazine's 2004 Book of the Year Awards

Publisher: Hatherleigh Press 2007

Distributor: Random House

"A sensitive topic ever so elegantly handled."

—**JUDITH COCHE, Ph.D.,** clinical psychologist, director, the Coche Center
Philadelphia, Pennsylvania

*   *   *

"Written with humoristic and didactic brilliance."

—**FRANK PEREZ-RIVAS, M.D.,** retired director, Oakland Park Veterans
Administration Clinic, Oakland Park, Florida

*   *   *

"This book takes the mystique out of heart disease and answers sex-related
questions that a patient might be too embarrassed to ask in person.
Chapunoff doesn't hold back on the humor—not a bad idea, considering
the gravity under which some readers might be studying this book. This
text has the potential for becoming a well-thumbed reference book."

—**KARL KUNKEL,** critic, *ForeWord Magazine*

*   *   *

"An intriguing, comfortable, and witty format to address intimate health issues. There are no other books addressing the issues he covers. Dr. Chapunoff has opened the door to a long-neglected subject. He is honest and forthright with his answers. This excellent resource proves that an informative and educational reading experience can also be engaging even when the subject matter is very serious."

—**BETTY CORBIN TUCKER,** author of *The Thorn of Sexual Abuse*, conductor of writing seminars

*   *   *

"In *Answering Your Questions*, Dr. Chapunoff examines the question of heart disease and sex from every angle—both medical and personal. The information is timely, thoroughly researched, and highly relevant. The author provides a knowledgeable and caring approach to an important new topic. Highly recommended!"

—**RAYMOND C. ROSEN, Ph.D.,** professor of psychiatry and medicine, Robert Wood Johnson Medical School, NJ; director of Human Sexuality Program; past president of the International Academy of Sex Research

*   *   *

"Any literate individual with an interest in his or her health and specifically anyone who wants to know more about love, life, hearts, sex, compassion, and human relationships will find this book of enormous value. Professionals can also derive benefit from Dr. Chapunoff's vast experience and profound wisdom. It makes me feel with all my heart that Dr. Chapunoff was my personal physician."

—**ARNOLD A. LAZARUS, Ph.D.,** distinguished professor emeritus of psychology, Rutgers University

*   *   *

"A special cardiologist offers an extraordinary guide for all who worry about life after heart disease. A provocative sense of humor makes the reading fun. I have not seen a more inspiring and integrative work on the connections between health, intimacy, and happiness. This book is a true celebration of the enduring human heart and spirit!"

—**SCOTT E. BORRELLI, Ed.D.**, collegiate professor, the University of Maryland, European Division; director of counseling services, the American Intercontinental University of London; chief editor of the *European* journal the EMDR practitioner (www.emdr-practitioner.net)

*   *   *

"Dr. Chapunoff's superb book is long overdue and a godsend for the sixty-three million Americans who have cardiovascular disease.

"With its easy-to-understand writing style, its poignant clinical vignettes, its solid medical advice, and a superb index, this book deserves to be widely read and recommended."

—**ALINE ZOLDBROD, Ph.D.**, author of *Sex Smart—ForeWord Magazine* award winner

*   *   *

"Filled with amusing anecdotes and intricate explanations, this book is of value to anyone who has a sex drive and a beating heart."

—**JACQUELINE SOUSA**, editor, *Coral Gables Living* magazine, Florida

*   *   *

"*Answering Your Questions About Heart Disease and Sex* is a fun, interesting read, employing a lot of humor and great anecdotes. And it's got to be a more fun and relevant read for a cardiac patient than the week-old *Better Homes and Gardens* in the hospital room. Forget the $20 get-well bouquet; give your convalescent a sex life for $15.95."

—**JOHN HUETTE,** book reviewer, *Boca Raton News*, Florida

*   *   *

"Dr. Eduardo Chapunoff is that rare learned man of science who takes a quintessentially worrisome, life-threatening, taboo-laced, and universally avoided subject such as sex and its ramifications to cardiac disease sufferers and offers them the balm of simple clarity, compassion, and rock-solid guidance. There's a reason Dr. Chapunoff is held in such high regard—his skill, his writing, and his guidance are totally approachable, gentle, and wise."

—**BERNIE AHEARN,** radio host, "A Man's World," Detroit, Michigan

* * *

"I liked this book. It was informative without being preachy, straightforward, and not so technical that it went over my head. By discussing things in a straightforward manner, readers will find there is little to be embarrassed about. Humor is generously sprinkled throughout to assist in this process."

—**NANCY GAIL,** BC Books, Georgia

* * *

"Upbeat, direct, straightforward, conversational style. Dr. Chapunoff is a master of knowing how to pull in his readers by presenting information that is current and relevant."

—**NORM GOLDMAN,** editor and publisher of *Books for Pleasure*, Montreal, Canada

DEDICATION

This book is dedicated to Mount Sinai Medical Center, Miami Beach, and its CEO Steven Sonenreich whose brilliant leadership has been truly inspiring.

Years ago, when I had my medical practice in Miami Beach, I belonged to the center's medical staff for twenty-five years. Taking care of critically ill patients with the total support of the institution's administrators and distinguished professional colleagues was a most rewarding and unforgettable experience.

Steven's humanity and administrative talent resulted in a medical center that is among the best in the world.

A number of years have passed since I was an attending physician at Mount Sinai but the institution's support of my practice, its humanity, and its excellence in the field of health care left an indelible mark and a profound gratitude that will last for the rest of my life, and beyond.

Eduardo Chapunoff, M.D., F.A.C.P., F.A.C.C.

ACKNOWLEDGMENTS

I want to express my deep appreciation to my wife Maria Cristina for her devotion, love, and understanding.

I am indebted to Drs. Robert T. Marema and Carlos Carrasquilla for contributing their expert opinions on morbid obesity and its surgical management and Mrs. Ileana Muniz whose courage and humanity allowed us to relate her personal experience in chapter 14 of this publication.

LIST OF FIGURES

PREFACE

There are different reasons that spark the initiative to write a book.

What did it this time was the observation of morbidly obese patients enjoying the results of their weight-loss surgery and those suffering from morbid obesity who were unable to shake the needle of the scale that kept on displaying an unmovable, recalcitrant mark.

It is easy for health care practitioners to urge obese patients to follow a diet and do regular exercises. It is a different story for patients to be able or willing to comply with these commendable recommendations. Some adhere to the instructed calories but, for a number of reasons—physical, psychological, or just simple boredom—are unable to do more walking or any kind of physical activity. Others will go through the efforts of exercise, but their food temptations remain difficult to resist.

Many who suffer from morbid obesity try to overcome the problem by making some lifestyle changes, such as reducing a little of their fats and carbohydrates consumption and walking a bit more three times a week. The trouble with this approach is that it doesn't work. When a person carries over one hundred pounds of excess weight—some people carry three hundred pounds of excess weight and occasionally more—normalizing the weight is a challenge of monumental proportions.

The formula for success—and by success I mean the achievement and preservation of the desirable weight—contains an essential ingredient, and that is *radical behavior modification.*

So this much is clear: regardless of the chosen therapeutic approach—conservative, (medical) or invasive (weight-loss surgery)—to produce and preserve good results, a person's behavior must change. It has to be not only different. It's got to be better. And I don't mind calling that change "revolutionary." Mild or casual modifications will not succeed. *The commitment to achieve long-lasting correction of morbid obesity must be decisive, consistent, and permanent.*

The causes of morbid obesity vary from person to person: genes, environment, behavior, insufficient physical activity, some illnesses, certain medications, and others contribute in an individual manner to each person's weight. The medical consequences of obesity and the risks posed by this disorder are not the same for all those affected. Some individuals are more vulnerable than others.

The above implies that the treatment approach toward all morbidly obese patients cannot be the same. Some patients—very few, indeed—will respond to diet and exercise. Others will require weight-loss surgery. The trouble is that many of them are not willing or able to do the former; and due to medical, psychological, psychiatric, or other reasons do not qualify for the latter.

Throughout the course of this book, I emphasize the critical contribution of morbid obesity to numerous illnesses although I placed more emphasis on complications affecting the cardiovascular system.

If you ever feel you're wasting your time becoming familiar with technical-medical knowledge, reverse that opinion immediately and get down to the business of learning what's going on in the field of obesity and its associated ailments. It is that knowledge that will make you grasp the immensity of the problem that affects you and, most significantly, the importance of correcting it.

I hope that something positive will come out of the criticism of some insurance corporation's attitudes toward patients who need quick and effective treatment and are often deprived of both. Many obese patients are left behind and do not receive adequate treatment because of insurance coverage problems, limitations, and exclusions. When dealing with morbid obesity, procrastination may cause a tragedy. I think the time is ripe to expand the discussion on this issue and come up with practical and badly needed solutions.

I do want to make one point clear: this book does not endorse obesity surgery for every individual who carries one hundred pounds or more of weight excess. For a number of reasons that will become clear as you read this book, this kind of treatment should be reserved for those who qualify for it. But what I am categorically suggesting is that when it is clear that a patient badly needs the operation because a medical evaluation indicates that he or she could become disabled or dead unless the procedure is carried out, weight-loss surgery should not be denied, and the paperwork that leads to its approval should not be delayed or obstructed, most particularly because of limitations imposed by economic calculations and miscalculations of some corporate executives who are far more concerned about their companies' profits than the well-being and survival of their clients.

At the end of this work, I describe the role of the American Society for Metabolic and Bariatric Surgery (ASMBS) and the Surgical Review Corporation (SRC). Thanks to these distinguished organizations and the guidance they provide to patients, health care professionals, and health insurance corporations in the United States and the rest of the world, many people are saved, painful illnesses go into remission, lives become more productive, and legions of patients no longer will become disabled or dead because of untreated complications of morbid obesity. The ASMBS and the SRC offer a list of Centers of Excellence. This category is only reserved for those who earned it with hard work, talent, and dedication.

I have a deep desire, and you feel free to categorize it as an ambition, if you wish: if only one person suffering from morbid obesity becomes healthier and happier and avoids a catastrophic outcome from this disease from reading this book, this publication will be totally justified.

Eduardo Chapunoff, Miami, 2010

INTRODUCTION

APPROACH TO MORBID OBESITY REALISM, HOPE, AND DETERMINATION

Some dreams turn into realities. The successful treatment of obesity is one of them.

Life is beautiful although, as we all know, it isn't always easy. Most of us want to enjoy healthy, peaceful, productive, and happy lives. Sometimes, intercepting developments disrupt the achievement of these desirable projections. Obesity is an example.

And it isn't just the numerous medical complications of obesity that make this condition so disturbing, but the psychological consequences, social and employment limitations, the discrimination and stigmatization it triggers as well as its frequent physical and emotional contribution to sexual dysfunctions.

Morbidly obese persons are sometimes perceived as weak willed, self-indulgent, ugly, and awkward. Even members of the medical profession (physicians, medical trainees, medical students, nurses, psychologists, counselors) are prejudiced about obese individuals.

This deplorable behavior sometimes leads to depression, social isolation, and substance abuse. Adults would rather miss both hands, be blind, deaf, or have ugly facial scars than be obese. College students stated that they would rather marry embezzlers, shoplifters, or cocaine users than obese persons.

Not all of those affected by severe obesity find it easy to accept it.

I once examined a thirty-four-year-old lady who carried 120 pounds of weight excess, and we had this exchange:

Dr. Chapunoff (Dr. C.): Alice, I made some calculations and concluded that you carry 120 pounds of weight excess. Would you like to do something about your obesity?

Alice (A): What obesity?

Dr. C.: I'm referring to your excessive weight.

A: I don't think I'm overweight. And I certainly wouldn't define myself as *obese*. Why do you call me *obese*?

Dr. C.: Well, with all due respect . . . medically, *morbid obesity* is defined as "a weight excess of one hundred pounds or more."

A: You can say and calculate anything you want, but I do not consider myself obese. And to be perfectly honest, I don't like the way *you* look!

Dr. C.: Oh, I see . . . Will you please tell me what's wrong with me?

A: Yeah, I'll tell you, you're too slim. You look like you need to eat a huge pepperoni pizza.

Dr. C: I do . . . ?

A: Yeah . . . and what do you plan to do about it?

Dr. C.: Nothing much, really, I'm satisfied the way I am. Oh, Alice, by the way, I love pepperoni pizza!

A: Me too! Dr. C [*with tears in her eyes*], I'm really happy the way I look too . . .

Dr. C.: That's fine. And remember, I never said that you don't look well. The point I am trying to make is not cosmetic but medical. Severe obesity is associated with cardiovascular disease, diabetes, high blood cholesterol levels, cancer, and a host of other illnesses.

A: I'm not convinced. Some relatives of mine are big, really extra-large-size people, and they are as strong as a horse.

DR. C.: Perhaps you need more information on the subject and the potential harm you could do to yourself. Now let me ask you a candid question. If you don't call 120 pounds of weight excess obesity, how would you define that situation?

A: OK, well . . . I'd say I'm a girl with a "little heavy frame."

DR. C.: All right, Alice, let me suggest you this. Think about my recommendations to do something about your weight. If you feel I can help you, call me back. I'll be happy to advise you further. How is that?

A: That's fine, Dr. Chapunoff. I promise you, I'll think about it.

DR. C.: There you go! Have a great day!

A: You too, Doctor.

Was this denial, wounded pride, self-image distortion, or something else?

Others offer different explanations:

I admitted to the hospital a forty-two-year-old four-hundred-pound gentleman in critical condition due to clots in the lungs that had traveled from the legs (acute pulmonary emboli). Obesity predisposes to this condition. Fortunately, he recovered. When I asked him what he thought about the possible origin of his obesity, he told me, "Food is the only thing in this world I have control on." His wife divorced him, his friends deserted him, business relationships and his financial base went sour.

And then, there are patients who are cheerful and positive, like a thirty-three-year-old female who carried one hundred pounds of weight excess, happy as anyone can be and "without emotional conflicts" who "didn't really eat much at all," exercised regularly (her powerful muscular development clearly proved that), but had a family history of morbid obesity (mother, aunts, sisters, brothers). So her genes, evidently, had a lot to do with her weight problem.

A DISEASE CALLED OBESITY

Obesity is a chronic, serious disease that results from a complex interaction of behavioral, environmental, and genetic factors, the end result of an imbalance between energy intake and energy expenditure.

FACTORS THAT CONTRIBUTE TO OBESITY

Advanced age associated with disabilities that lead to physical inactivity.

Ethnic-racial. In the United States, obesity occurs at higher rates in certain minorities populations such as African Americans, Hispanic Americans, and the American Indians. Asian Americans have a relatively low prevalence for obesity.

Sixty-six percent of African American women, 66 percent of Mexican American women, and 49 percent of Caucasian women are overweight.

Gender. For women, the black population has the highest prevalence of overweight (78 percent) and obesity (50.8 percent).

For men, the Mexican American population has the highest prevalence of overweight (74.4 percent) and obesity (29.4 percent).

Note: A person is considered overweight when the body mass index (BMI) is greater than or equal to twenty-five and obese when the BMI is greater or equal to thirty. Morbid obesity is a BMI greater or equal to forty. The BMI is a formula that calculates the person's weight in relation to his or her height.

Socioeconomic status. Excessive weight affects African Americans (men and women) of all socioeconomic levels. Minority women with low income appear to have the greatest likelihood of being overweight.

In the United States, the trend is to consume more sugars and fats. The reasons have been thought to be largely economic.

Energy-dense foods rich in sugar and fat are the cheapest. Dr. Adam Drewnowski, director of Nutritional Sciences Program in the UW School of Public Health and Community Medicine stated that *"as long as the healthier lean meats, fish, and fresh produce remain more expensive, obesity will continue to be a problem for the working poor."*

Corrective recommendations include weight-reducing diets that poor people cannot afford. Dr. Drewnowski adds the following: *"Whereas obesity affects minorities and the poor, most of our suggested remedies are resolutely middle class."*

Genes are important. Adopted children resemble more closely to their biological parents than to their adoptive parents.

African American women of similar income and education were observed to remain more than twice as likely to be obese than European American women.

Pima Indians obesity is also thought to have a significant genetic component. Pima Indians are known as one of the heaviest groups of people in the world. Some adults weigh more than five hundred pounds.

Food industry. Diets around the globe are shaped by large food industrial corporations that consider profits—not public health—their main objective. They constantly battle to increase demands and sales.

Globalization has affected the way people eat. Agricultural, food, and retail companies have consolidated into large international corporations. A handful of huge organizations control the food market. The public passively absorbs the propaganda and enjoys the taste of foods saturated with fats, carbohydrates, salt, and large-serving size that sell at a cheaper price so people may consume more of them. Take an example: the chicken. Consumption of chicken has risen by more than 1,000 percent in the past fifty years in the United States. Chickens are now genetically programmed to reach market weight in as little as forty days. This is done by the chemical manipulation of feeding, hormones, and antibiotics.

Corrective action should address

*   corporate behavior: advertisement often includes misleading ads;
*   insufficient information on healthy eating;
*   massive production of unhealthy foods needs international regulation;
*   in certain places, such as schools, lots of items should be prohibited.

Alcohol has seven calories per gram. These are "empty" calories because alcohol contains no beneficial nutrients, such as vitamins and minerals.

A twelve-ounce beer contains about 150 calories. Sugary, carbonated beverages and fruit juices contribute additional calories when mixed with alcohol in a cocktail. A twelve-ounce beer, a five-ounce glass of wine, and a 1.5-ounce shot of liquor have about the same amount of alcohol and equivalent caloric content. Alcohol is a significant source of calories, and drinking usually stimulates eating, particularly in social settings.

Cultural. Fatness has traditionally been a great concern in Western societies. There are cultural stereotypes of attractiveness, and it is difficult for some to go against the socially accepted trends. In many instances, eating disorders appear to be linked to cultural standards.

Young people seem to be particularly vulnerable to social pressures. When a heavier weight is socially favored, food consumption increases. Conversely, teenagers who have equated popularity with thinness are candidates to suffer from anorexia. They resort to extreme measures such as vomiting and dangerous medications. If weight control is not achieved, peer pressure becomes intolerable.

The American environment encourages people to eat. Wherever you go, there's food waiting for you. Bad eating habits are contagious and hard to control. Watching a pal enjoying food represents a temptation difficult to resist.

Years ago, I was invited to an all-Argentine barbecue party. I was born and raised in Argentina. Beef and sausages are a very important part of that country's diet. Everyone was supposed to bring his own meal. Since all the guests were from Argentina, they wanted to enjoy the food they like the best, namely, steaks and sausages. But I wanted to be different. I wanted to be the guy who knew better, who was able to sacrifice the delicious taste of a traditional steak for a piece of salmon that projected health and virtuous eating habits.

So I took to the party a salmon steak. There were guys standing close to the fire, each one cooking his own meat. I unfolded my salmon piece and displayed it like a trophy. I was so proud of it!

But then, the smell of the burning beef drove me nuts. I quickly decided that I had to disrupt my low cholesterol diet, put it on hold, and enjoy the steak. I offered to trade off my salmon cut for a beefsteak, but nobody was willing to eat the fish.

Finally, someone felt sorry for me and threw into my plate a steak that—needless to say—I voraciously ate.

We are all human, we have weaknesses, and we make mistakes. An occasional dietary sin may not matter that much, but repetitive deviations of your carefully drafted nutritional program is the wrong way to go and will eventually cause problems.

Smoking cessation. The average weight gain after quitting smoking is six to eight pounds. Ten percent of people who stop smoking gain thirty pounds or more. Quitting smoking increases a person's appetite and a tendency to have more snacks and alcoholic drinks. Diet and exercise will do the trick.

Prolonged inactivity. I had a patient who sustained serious legs injuries and required multiple surgeries to his lower extremities. He was bedridden for eleven years. His weight was around seven hundred pounds. That didn't stop him from having a serious relationship with his girlfriend for a number of years (she was very attractive and her weight was normal).

Religion. A 1998 study (Ferraro) found that states with large numbers of persons professing a religious affiliation had higher than average numbers of obese people.

Whereas 1 percent or less of those embracing the Jewish, Muslim, Hindu, Buddhist, or other non-Christian religious qualify as obese, the numbers of the markedly obese rise dramatically among various Christian denominations (17 percent to 27 percent).

Two reasons are suspected of being responsible for this phenomenon:

* Non-Christian religions have some dietary restrictions. Protestant faiths, for the most part, do not.
* Christian religious environments seem to have frequent postsermon coffee and pastry gatherings, potluck dinners, church picnics, pancake breakfast fund-raisers, and Sunday sundae socials are common traditional activities.

Pregnancy. Obesity is one of the most frequent causes for complications in pregnancy. The mother is considered obese if at the beginning of her pregnancy her BMI is over twenty-five.

Weight gain during pregnancy depends on the following:

- The mother's weight at the beginning of pregnancy
- Genes
- Excessive eating during pregnancy
- Reduced physical activity
- The weight of the fetus
- The size of the placenta
- The amount of amniotic fluid
- Fluid retention

An obese pregnant woman is at a greater risk of contracting hypertension and diabetes.

Menopause. Decline of estrogen production plus physical inactivity leads to weight gain in postmenopausal women and contribute to myocardial infarctions, hypertension, and diabetes. Weight loss may reverse some of these complications. Lifestyle changes are essential.

Dietary habits. Many become established in childhood. If you want a child to learn to eat right, give him/her healthy food as soon as he/she has the ability to put food into his/her mouth.

Hormonal disorders. Examples: *Hypothyroidism*—"a deficient production of thyroid hormone." *Hypothalamic dysfunction* that leads to overeating (the hypothalamus is a vital part of the brain that regulates body temperature, metabolic and other important activities). *Adrenal gland disorders* that produce excessive amounts of cortisone. *A pancreatic tumor called insulinoma*: excessive production of insulin by this tumor causes frequent hypoglycemia and the need for frequent eating.

History of Gestational Diabetes.

Oral contraceptives. Some women gain weight when taking the pill (5.0 to 6.6 pounds after one year of contraception). This may be due to fluid retention or increased appetite.

How could one minimize weight gain? By using the lowest possible estrogen containing birth control pill. Current twenty microgram pills, which are the lowest estrogen doses available, are Alesse, Levlite, Loestrin Fe, Mircette.

Medications. Contraceptives, antiretroviral therapy, antiseizure medications (valproic acid), antipsychotics, insulin, steroids (cortisone derivatives), oral antidiabetic agents.

Antidepressants. Elavil, Sinequan, Paxil, Prozac, Effexor, Zoloft, Celexa, Cymbalta, Lexapro.

Buspar has been associated with weight loss.

Patients who prematurely discontinue the antidepressant as a result of increased appetite or weight gain may fall back into depression.

Tube feeding. Patients who are not able to swallow food are fed through a feeding tube placed in the stomach by an abdominal incision. If excessive amount of calories is provided and the physical activity is markedly reduced, the result is weight gain.

Polycystic ovarian syndrome. This disorder presents menstrual irregularities, excessive hair growth in various parts of the body (hirsutism), acne, a male pattern of baldness, and increased blood androgen levels. The mechanisms that lead to obesity are complex.

Prolactinoma. This is a pituitary gland tumor with a high prevalence of weight gain.

And other disorders that will not be mentioned here.

OBESITY AS A DISEASE ENTITY

The dangers of obesity were recognized over two thousand years ago by Hippocrates. He is widely recognized as the father of medicine. He died in the year 361 BC, at the age of ninety-nine. Some of this great Greek physician's aphorisms persisted for generations. Here is one of them: *"Fat persons are more exposed to sudden death than the slender."*

It took longer than twenty-two centuries for the medical science to prove him correct.

Obesity wasn't classified as a disease until 1985 when the National Institutes of Health held a Consensus Development Conference on the health implications of obesity. That was a historic event. Experts concluded that obesity is a *serious chronic disease associated with a number of associated illnesses called comorbidities* (hypertension, diabetes, high levels of cholesterol, obstructive sleep apnea, heart attacks, etc.) *that lead to excess mortality.*

A Veterans Administration study of two hundred morbidly obese men aged twenty-three to seventy years, with an average weight of 316 pounds, showed a twelvefold increase in mortality in the twenty-five- to thirty-four-year age group and a sixfold increase in the thirty-five- to forty-four-year age group.

If you want to see examples of morbid obesity contributing to premature obituaries, see the *Guinness World Records*. None of the heaviest people on the planet lived over forty years of age.

It has also been observed that a 20 percent increase in body weight or more constitutes a health hazard. Conversely, even a 10 percent weight reduction positively influences a person's health.

Defining obesity as a disease carries more than academic implications. The economic issues at stake are complex, and there are no easy solutions. The estimated annual cost of obesity in the United States is $117 billion. The cost of lost productivity due to obesity represents approximately $4 billion annually.

THE OBESITY EPIDEMIC

Approximately 127 million adult Americans are overweight; nine million of those suffer from morbid obesity. A morbidly obese person is one who carries one hundred or more pounds of weight excess.

The Centers for Disease Control and Prevention (CDC)—1999-2000—estimated that 64 percent of U.S. adults are either overweight (33 percent) or obese (31 percent). The extremely obese (BMI > forty) represents 4.7 percent of the population.

Other countries are showing similar trends. The incidence of obesity in Europe is 10-20 percent for men and 10-25 percent for women. The most shocking increase has occurred in England where the prevalence of obesity doubled between 1980 and 1995. In Japan, obesity has doubled among men in the last twenty years and almost doubled for young women. In China, obesity is more common in urban areas and among women.

A great concern is the rapid rise in numbers of overweight and obese children and adolescents. Approximately, 20-25 percent of children are either overweight or obese. Boys and girls are equally affected.

Developing countries in Asia and the Middle East (Saudi Arabia, Egypt, Jordan, Lebanon), Central and South America are also having considerable increase in obesity.

There are at least 250 million obese people in the world (7 percent of the world population).

The tendency in the United States is toward an increase of one pound per year after age twenty-five. Since the muscle and bone mass decrease with age, the fat increase is actually a gain of one and a half pound per year. Therefore, by age fifty-five, the average American has added about thirty-seven pounds of fat during the course of adulthood.

Environmental and behavioral factors are mainly to blame. The portions of high-calorie foods have increased substantially. Four decades ago, a soda contained eight ounces. Nowadays, the size is thirty-two ounces. A double cheeseburger with french fries and a Coke provide you with enough calories to spend the whole winter in underwear at the North Pole. Long hours of watching television, the Internet, and computer games have a lot to do with children's, teenagers', and adults' excessive weight.

In the United States, only 22 percent of adults and 25 percent of adolescents engage in significant regular physical activity.

THE PRICE OF ADVANCED TECHNOLOGY

Modern life and technological advances have promoted obesity by decreasing expenditure of energy. Machines have replaced muscles; cranes substituted arms and legs. Cars and buses facilitate transportation and often require prolonged sitting. The same applies to those who drive their own cars to their jobs. The drive-through is use to pick up medications at a pharmacy or shirts at the dry-cleaning store or food or do a banking transaction.

Thirty percent of obese patients have eating disorders, and it is important for the health care practitioner to screen for them when taking the patient's history: food-seeking behavior, lack of satiety, purging, binging. Obsessive-compulsive disorders and anxiety may lead to obesity and so does depression with self-destructive inclinations. Depression is often associated with marked reduction in physical activity.

THE SCALE MAKES A POINT: WHAT'S TO BE DONE NEXT?

Correction of obesity requires motivation, method, and perseverance. Casual approaches are useless. A positive attitude makes a big difference. Feelings of deception and frustration are taxing and burdensome. Do not allow them to intimidate you. Try this formula: *Don't hate the problem. Instead, love the challenge!*

Tough times lie ahead? Of course! But instead of saying, "Oh my god, how am I going to deal with all this?" Say, "I'm overcoming my problems one by one. Come on, little bastards, come into my life. I will dispose of you with my bright outlook, my faith, my sense of purpose, and my great reservoir of optimism."

DIET AND EXERCISE VERSUS WEIGHT-LOSS SURGERY (WLS), ALSO CALLED BARIATRIC SURGERY (BS)

Most weight-loss management medical programs are ineffective. The best weight-loss programs achieve about 10 percent of body weight loss, but patients usually regain two-thirds of the weight loss within a year and regain almost all of it within five years.

Complications of weight-loss surgery (WLS) may occur—and do occur—at the best hospitals, with the best anesthesiologists, the best surgeons, and the best nursing care. Other variables play pivotal roles—medical illnesses and pulmonary or heart disease.

WLS as a possible treatment should be considered when

1. **you have not responded to medical management, diet, and exercise;**
2. **your obesity and associated illnesses carry higher risk of disability and death than the risks of WLS;**
3. **you have access to an experienced and skillful obesity surgeon and health care team;**

4. you are psychologically ready for a radical change in behavior on permanent basis that will require eating limitations, regular exercise, and medical follow-up for the rest of your life.

So it isn't really a matter of being in favor or against WLS. You should only be in favor of what is right for you. If you can solve the problem by diet and exercise, you should not even think about WLS. On the other hand, if conscientious efforts on your part have failed and your clinical evaluation projects great likelihood for strokes, heart attacks, heart failure, disabling or fatal illnesses, then you start considering WLS as a viable option.

THE SELECTION OF A SURGEON

The prevalence of severe obesity has been increasing at an alarming rate. Not surprisingly, more surgeons are performing weight-loss surgery.

Skillfully done, weight-loss surgery (WLS) can be one of the most rewarding experiences in the practice of the medical profession—for both the doctor and the patient—but suboptimally performed, complications multiply; and a valuable operation gets an unfair reputation.

Patients who are definite candidates for bariatric surgery are advised by their health providers *against* it when their experience on this field is practically nonexistent. So patients *often do not have enough information* about the hazards of morbid obesity and the state-of-the-art operations currently available to correct it. *Or worse than that, they have the wrong information.*

If it is apparent that diet and exercise produced no meaningful results and knowledgeable specialists concluded that *medically and psychologically* you do, indeed, qualify for weight-loss surgery, select the best possible surgeon, assisted by the best possible team, at the best possible hospital.

Bear in mind that, ultimately, *you are in charge* of your life. Your physician, a surgeon, a psychologist, a friend, this book, another book *may help you to understand what morbid obesity is, what it means, and how it can be managed; but you, and only you, will have to confront the challenge, draw a conclusion, and make a decision.*

It is then that you'll do whatever you think is best for you, and with all the hope and faith in the world that things will turn out the right way.

CHAPTER 1

COMORBIDITIES: MORBID OBESITY'S DANGEROUS PALS

The good news about complications of obesity is that many of them can be prevented or dramatically improved by substantial weight-loss achievement.

Obesity wasn't discovered yesterday. What has been recognized relatively recently—approximately three decades ago—is the important relationship between obesity and disease.

Obesity causes harm by itself and by its association with other conditions that frequently coexist with it. These are called comorbidities. We'll soon see what they are and what they mean.

OBESITY: WHAT IS IT?

Obesity is an excess of total body fat that results from an imbalance created by an abnormally high caloric intake that is not matched by a corresponding increase in energy expenditure. *Obesity exists when there's an excessive percentage of body fat in relation to the percentage of muscular tissue.*

Individuals with great muscular development may carry higher than normal weight and are not considered obese. Why? Because they have a low percentage of body fat. Others who have normal or even under normal weight may have excessive body fat, typically located in the abdomen. Therefore, *an individual may be overweight due to excellent muscular development and not be obese while another who is underweight may have abdominal obesity.*

HOW TO MEASURE OBESITY

There are simple and sophisticated methods to measure obesity.

The currently most accepted and frequently used measurement in medical practice to express the degree of obesity is the *body mass index (BMI)*. This is calculated by a formula that includes the person's weight in relation to his or her height.

	BMI	Approximate pounds overweight
Underweight	under 18.5	
Normal	18.6-24.9	0
Overweight	25.0-26.9	1-20
OBESITY		
Mild	27.0-27.9	20-50
Moderate	30.0-34.9	50-75
Severe	35.0-39.9	75-100
Morbid	40.0-49.9	100-200
Super Morbid	50.0-60.0	200+

For men, waist circumferences greater than 94 centimeters (over 80 centimeters in women) increase the potential for cardiovascular risk. Circumferences greater than 102 centimeters for men and more than eighty-eight centimeters for women require urgent medical intervention.

OBESITY WORKS IN THE SHADOWS

Obesity causes disease by acting surreptitiously for years. Then one day and not necessarily at the most convenient time, the alarm goes off.

Obese individuals experience complex cellular, chemical, and vascular reactions that unnoticeably—and incessantly—take place inside their bodies. This goes on until an acute medical event occurs and an ambulance rushes the victim to a hospital's Emergency Department. Common events are myocardial infarction, congestive heart failure, stroke, a life-threatening arrhythmia, pulmonary emboli, or a cardiac arrest.

It was previously thought that obesity causes harm *because of its association* with conditions such as diabetes, hypertension, lipids abnormalities, and other comorbidities. In the past several years, evidence that strongly suggests that *obesity per se is a significant cardiac risk factor has been accumulating*. Some studies have shown that minimal increases in a person's body mass index (BMI) are associated with higher risk of both nonfatal and fatal heart attacks *even if the person does not have other risk factors for heart disease*. Conversely, weight reduction appears to reduce the risk of heart attacks and heart failure.

You've probably never considered morbid obesity a disease because it never gave you "real problems." But *obesity is an ongoing disease even if you feel well, and the condition is not causing any symptoms or visible damage of any kind*.

The best way to prevent complications of a disease is, obviously, not having it. If you want to be a winner, catch the ball before it touches the ground. Get rid of your excessive weight *before* a serious complication occurs.

LIFE EXPECTANCY

Obesity is associated with a significant reduction in life expectancy for both men and women. This risk has been observed to be greater in overweight adults aged twenty to forty-four years than in those aged forty-five to seventy-four years. There is also increased incidence of early sudden death. This is doubled compared to nonobese individuals.

The risk of death from diabetes or heart attack is five to seven times greater.

BODY FAT DISTRIBUTION: UPPER AND LOWER OBESITY

Upper body obesity (abdominal obesity), also called android obesity, is more strongly associated with high blood pressure, cholesterol, blood clotting abnormalities, diabetes, and cardiovascular death than lower body obesity (gluteal adiposity predominance), also called gynoid obesity. Here, the fat is preferentially localized in the gluteofemoral regions (buttocks and thighs).

COMORBIDITIES

Conditions frequently associated with obesity and are commonly known as *obesity-related illnesses (comorbidities)*.

Hypertension is three to five times more likely to occur in obese than in nonobese individuals, high cholesterol levels twice more, diabetes three times more likely, and endometrial cancer five times more likely.

The list of obesity-associated conditions is a long one, as you'll see a few lines below.

One suggestion: do not go over the comorbidities list too quickly. *Take your time to read them and think about them and visualize how much physical and psychological suffering they can inflict.* As a rule, several of them coexist in the same individual, and many organs are simultaneously affected.

DISEASES CLOSELY ASSOCIATED WITH MORBID OBESITY

1. Heart disease
2. Vascular disease (arteries)
3. Vascular disease (veins)
4. Disorders commonly associated with morbid obesity (diabetes, hypertension, blood lipids abnormalities)
5. Respiratory abnormalities
6. Gastrointestinal disease
7. Arthritis-orthopedic problems
8. Neurological disorders
9. Sleep disturbances
10. Renal failure
11. Hormonal disorders
12. Hypercoagulable states
13. Impaired immunity
14. Cancer
15. Accidents and traumas with delayed recoveries
16. Psychological dysfunctions
17. Psychiatric illnesses
18. Sexual dysfunction
19. Skin diseases
20. Propensity to wound infections
21. Urinary incontinence
22. Anal incontinence
23. Cataracts
24. Periodontitis
25. Metabolic syndrome

1. **HEART DISEASE**
   - **Atherosclerotic heart disease.** Disease of the coronary arteries. Fatty plaques deposits inside these vessels.
   - **Congestive heart failure.** The heart muscle becomes weak.
   - **Cardiomyopathy of obesity.** Invasion of fat into the heart muscle.
   - **Atrial fibrillation.** Rhythm disturbance caused by "shivering of the atrial muscle."
   - **Malignant life-threatening arrhythmias**

2. **VASCULAR DISEASE (ARTERIAL)**
   - **Strokes.** These result from either a blockage of a cerebral or carotid artery produced by a large atherosclerotic plaque, a clot, or both or rupture of a cerebral artery (cerebral hemorrhage).
   - **Peripheral arterial disease (PAD).** Occlusion of upper and lower extremities arteries or abdominal arteries.
   - **Aortic aneurysm**

3. **VASCULAR DISEASE (VENOUS)**
   - **Varicosities of lower extremities.** Diseased dilated veins with sluggish circulation.
   - **Venous ulcers and leg infections**
   - **Edema of lower extremities (fluid accumulation)**
   - **Phlebitis.** Painful inflammation of leg veins
   - **DVT (deep venous thrombosis).** Blood clots formed in the veins of the lower extremities.
   - **Lymphedema.** Chronic swelling of legs due to malfunction of lymphatic vessels.

4. **DISORDERS COMMONLY ASSOCIATED WITH MORBID OBESITY**
   - **Diabetes**
   - **Hypertension**
   - **Dyslipidemia**

   All of the above increase the incidence of cardiovascular disease.

5. **RESPIRATORY ABNORMALITIES**
   Upper airway obstruction (OSA or Obstructive sleep apnea)
   Lung disease
   - **Asthma** (bronchial spasms)
   - **Chronic bronchitis** (infection of the bronchial tree)
   - **Hypoventilation.** This is poor oxygen absorption and inadequate carbon dioxide elimination due to a mechanical

respiratory impairment. The added weight of the thoracic cage and abdomen due to excessive fatty tissue reduces the expansion of the chest walls and the lungs.

- **Pulmonary emboli** (clots that travel from the lower extremities [calves and thighs] and get lodged in the lungs)

6. GASTROINTESTINAL DISEASE

- **Gastroesophageal reflux disease (GERD).** Gastric juice moves into the esophagus causing heartburn and lower esophagus inflammation.
- **Inguinal and umbilical (nable) hernias**
- **Gallbladder stones** due to increased secretion of cholesterol in the bile
- **Fatty liver.** Accumulation of fat that causes steatohepatitis or fat-induced hepatitis. This is due to deposits of triglycerides in the liver cells in the form of fat droplets.
- **Pancreatitis.** High blood levels of triglycerides is associated with higher incidence of pancreas inflammation. This presents acute and severe abdominal pain.

7. ARTHRITIS AND ORTHOPEDIC PROBLEMS

- **More frequent involvement in knees and ankles (weight-bearing joints).** *The joints suffer the trauma of excessive weight. Lumbar spine and hips are affected too.*
- **Gout.** Inflammation of joints due to uric acid crystals accumulation.
- **Foot pain (heel) known as Sever's syndrome**
- **Hip pain and limping.** The head of the femur slips out of place
- **Blount disease.** Bowing of the tibia in preadolescents. Excessive weight exerts a downward pressure that is heavy enough to bend the leg bone.

The two major orthopedic complications of morbid obesity are the slipping of the femoral head and Blount's disease.

8. NEUROLOGICAL

- **Migraine**
- **Pseudotumor cerebri.** Condition associated with morbid obesity that causes headaches and impaired vision, including blindness. The mechanism is unknown. This disorder's symptoms resemble those of a brain tumor, but the patient does not have a brain tumor.
- **Carpal-tunnel syndrome.** Compression of the wrist's nerves.

9. SLEEP DISORDER
- **This is part of the sleep apnea syndrome (disturbed sleep plus snoring at night plus somnolence during the day).**

Note: If you ever have an interview with a severely obese person who might be an executive, a doctor, or an attorney, and he or she struggles to remain awake and dozes off until proven otherwise, that person suffers from sleep apnea.

10. RENAL FAILURE
- **Nephrotic syndrome.** Spilling of protein in the urine.
- **Nephrosclerosis.** Disease of multiple branches of renal arteries resulting from diabetes and/or hypertension that leads to shrinking of the kidneys and renal failure.

11. ENDOCRINOLOGICAL (HORMONAL) DISORDERS
- **Abnormal menses**
- **Infertility.** It can be corrected when morbid obesity is corrected.
- **Uterine fibroid tumors**
- **Polycystic ovaries**
- **Excessive blood levels of testosterone: facial hair, acne**
- **Dangerous effects of pregnancy:**
  - Hypertension
  - Gestational diabetes
  - C-section is required more frequently
  - Increased fetal mortality
  - Increased incidence of spina bifida in babies

12. HYPERCOAGULABLE STATES
Facilitate clot formation inside arteries and veins.

13. IMPAIRED IMMUNITY
Obesity decreases the body's resistance to harmful organisms.
There is a decrease activity of "scavenger" cells that destroy germs.

14. MALIGNANCIES (CANCER)
Both men and women with a BMI greater than forty have a higher incidence of death from cancer than normal weight subjects (BMI 18.5-24.9).

For both women and men: cancer of esophagus, colon, rectum, liver, gallbladder, pancreas, kidney, non-Hodgkin's lymphoma, multiple myeloma

For women: increased risk endometrial and cervical uterine, ovary, and breast cancer

For men: increased risk of stomach, colon-rectum, and prostate cancer

Breast cancer
Estrogens, which can promote breast cancer growth, are produced in excess amounts in obese women.

Steroid hormones are also increased in obesity and can trigger proliferation of malignant cells.

Breast cancer: this is the number 1 cancer linked with obesity and relates to it more than any other form of cancer.

Increased alcohol consumption may produce excess of estrogens and has been associated with increased risk of breast cancer.

Uterine cancer
The relationship between obesity and uterine cancer has been clearly established. Estrogens appear to be the culprit. These hormones induce characteristic heavy menstrual periods in obese women. Estrogens stimulate the inner layer of the uterus (endometrium), and that may result in endometrial cancer.

Prostate cancer
Prostate cancer is associated with aging and obesity. African American men have a significantly higher incidence of prostate cancer compared to that of white men.

Renal cancer
More so in obese women than in obese men.

Colon cancer
More so in obese men than in obese women.

Esophageal cancer
Gastroesophageal reflux commonly present in the morbidly obese is a risk factor for esophageal cancer.

15. ACCIDENTS AND TRAUMAS HAVE DELAYED RECOVERIES

16. PSYCHO-SOCIAL REACTIONS AND COMPLICATIONS
* Anxiety
* Depression (more prevalent in younger patients and women)
* Denial
* Poor self-esteem
* Self-loathing and sadness
* Insecurities
* Embarrassment
* Public disapproval
* Frustration
* Inability to sit on ordinary chairs
* Social stigmatization (rejection, prejudices)
* Discrimination (social and at the workplace)
* Negative impact on employment (affecting selection, placement, compensation, promotion)
* Difficulties in finding or keeping relationships

17. PSYCHIATRIC DISORDERS
* Bipolar
* Major depression
* Eating disorders
* Others

18. SEXUAL DYSFUNCTION
* Self-image problem, low self-esteem
* Relationship conflicts created by the existence of morbid obesity
* Comorbid conditions, such as hypertension, atherosclerosis, diabetes, or smoking (These are physical causes of sexual dysfunction.)
* Unpleasant odor due to difficulties in controlling hygiene (urine, fungal, and bacterial infections, persistent humidity in the groin and genital areas due to secretions of skin infections, excessive perspiration, and urinary incontinence)
* Difficulties in finding the genitals (a prominent abdomen hides the genitals and makes the contact of the hand with the penis difficult or impossible)
* Generalized weakness, fatigue, and shortness of breath due to excessive weight

* Difficulties for sexual intercourse with certain positions:
  - The severely obese patient may have shortness of breath lying flat on his or her back.
  - The male on top position is not tolerated by the woman due to the man's heavy weight exerting pressure on her thorax unless body-to-body contact is avoided.
  - The male on top position (missionary position) is difficult to tolerate by the male partner because his elbows placed on the bed must support the heavy body weight. This quickly translates into exhaustion.

19. SKIN DISEASES
* Skin bacterial and fungal infections
* Cellulitis
* Panniculitis (infected abdominal skin folds)
* Rashes
* Excessive perspiration
* Stretch marks (striae)
* Acanthosis nigricans (deepening pigmentation around the neck, axilla)
* Hirsutism (excessive hair growth) in women may result from increased production of testosterone, which is often associated with visceral obesity (accumulation of fat in various organs).

20. PROPENSITY TO WOUND INFECTIONS

21. URINARY INCONTINENCE

22. ANAL INCONTINENCE

23. CATARACTS

24. PERIODONTITIS (inflammation and infection of the gums and tissues surrounding the teeth)

25. THE METABOLIC SYNDROME
This entity represents a group of risk factors predictive of cardiovascular diseases and is the simultaneous presence of factors known to increase risk for developing type 2 diabetes and cardiovascular disease. It is also known as syndrome X and insulin resistant syndrome. *This diagnosis is made when three or more of the following five components are present:*

* A waist circumference greater than 102 centimeters for men and more than 88 centimeters for women.
* A fasting triglyceride level higher than 150 milligrams per deciliter
* A high-density lipoprotein (HDL) cholesterol level less than 40 milligrams per deciliter for men and less than 50 milligrams per deciliter for women
* Blood pressure higher than 135/80
* Fasting serum glucose concentration greater than 110 milligrams per deciliter

Obesity-related illnesses can be prevented, minimized, or resolved by eliminating the culprit: morbid obesity.

If you carry one hundred pounds or more of weight excess, *most likely, you already have some of the mentioned comorbidities, and there's a good probability that you are not aware of their existence.*

Morbid obesity affects many organs. In fact, one has trouble to find *any* organ or system in the human body that is not be affected by this disorder: the skin, eyes, joints, muscles, heart, arteries, veins, kidneys, stomach, esophagus, liver, brain, sexual organs, nervous system, and more are all targets for this destructive illness.

OBESITY-RELATED CONDITIONS THAT REQUIRE QUICK ATTENTION AND AGGRESSIVE TREATMENT APPROACH

* Pseudo-tumor cerebri: see bullet 9 above "Neurological"
* Type 2 diabetes
* Slipped femoral head: see bullet 7 above "Arthritis and orthopedic problems"
* Blount disease: bowing of the tibial bone in growing children. See bullet 7 above "Arthritis and orthopedic problems"
* Sleep apnea—see bullet 10 above—sleep disorders and chapter 4

The *successful treatment of morbid obesity* is followed by very substantial improvement or resolution of its numerous comorbidities, including most cases of pseudo-tumor cerebri, metabolic syndrome, polycystic ovarian syndrome, hirsutism, menstrual irregularities, asthma, type 2 diabetes, venous stasis disease, reflux esophagitis, hypertension, dyslipidemia, obstructive sleep apnea, nonalcoholic fatty liver disease, cardiovascular disease.

Also resolved or greatly improved are cases of stress urinary incontinence, gout, migraine, depression, and degenerative joint disease.

The quality of life improves in 95 percent of patients, and there's a five-year mortality reduction of 89 percent.

WHAT REALLY WORKS?

To succeed in the treatment of morbid obesity, radical behavior modification is essential. Unless you reach that point, no treatment for severe obesity, either medical or surgical, will work.

The best obesity center and the best surgeon in the world *will only help you* to correct the problem. *But only you* will have the key to success. *It will be your cooperation, your mental attitude as well as your mental fortitude, your permanent commitment to eat the right foods in the right amounts, the compliance with regular exercise, and a well-supervised medical follow-up that is going to turn your life around* and transform a potential nightmare, a tsunami wave of medical calamities, into a pleasant, healthy, and happy life, plentiful in beautiful projects and renewed opportunities.

CHAPTER 2

OBESITY AND HEART DISEASE
THE BELL RINGS:
MR. PROBLEM HAS ARRIVED!

Obesity and heart disease frequently coexist, and their association shouldn't take anybody by surprise. We should only get surprised by the unexpected.

Describing a medical subject to the general public is, in a way, like walking on a tight rope: a balance must be achieved between the explanation of technicalities and the appealing and didactic manner these need to be exposed.

It is certainly not a good idea to tell you that obesity may cause acute myocardial infarctions, heart failure, and strokes, without explaining what these conditions are. *Learning these concepts may change the way you think. Acting on them may change the way you live.*

Many errors in food consumption and lifestyles we make in the course of our lives cause illnesses and suffering that can be avoided by adopting preventive measures. When disease strikes, we ask ourselves, *How did that happen?* or *Why did that happen?* or *Did that have to happen?*

THE HEART AS A PUMP: HOW THE CARDIOVASCULAR SYSTEM WORKS

The heart and the circulatory system (arteries and veins) make up your *cardiovascular system.* Your heart is the pump that ejects blood to all the organs, tissues, and cells of the body.

The left ventricle ejects blood into the aorta, and the branches of this large artery supply oxygen and nutrients to all organs and tissues. The blood releases part of its oxygen during this process and becomes darker (venous blood). It is then collected by the venous system, which drains it into the right atrium and right ventricle. From here, this poorly oxygenated blood travels to the lungs where it absorbs oxygen, becomes fresh and fully oxygenated again, moves to the left atrium through the pulmonary veins, passes into the left ventricle, and is ejected into the aorta and the arterial tree, starting a new cycle.

Figure 1. Important Parts of the Heart

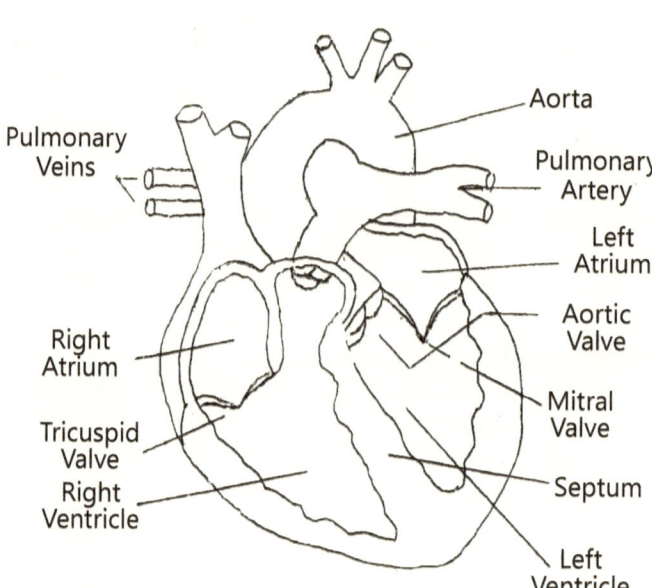

Figure 2. The Arterial Circulation

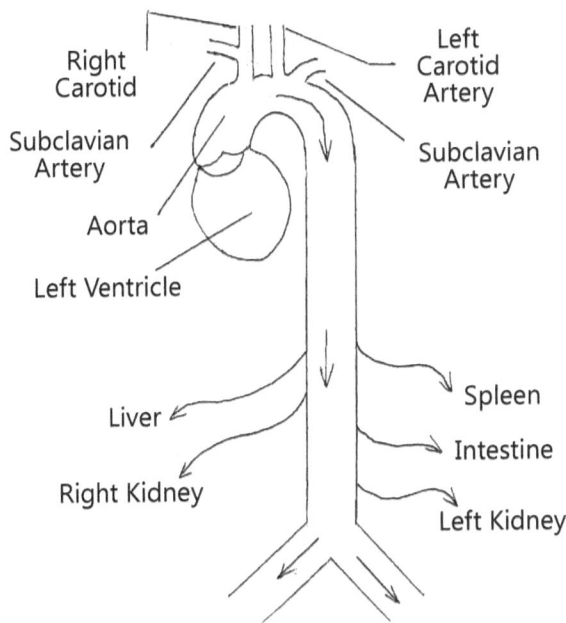

**The left ventricle ejects oxygenated blood into the aorta.
Aorta's multiple branches distribute blood throughout the body.**

Figure 3. Venous circulation drains blood into the right side of the heart.

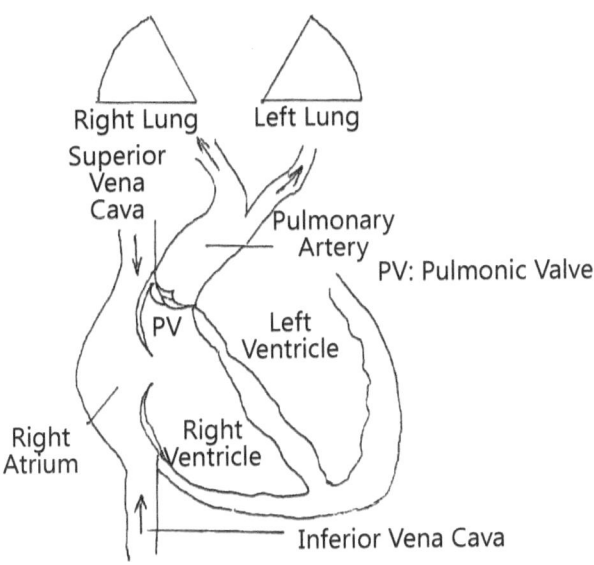

After arterial blood is supplied to all tissues and organs, it is collected by the venous system and drained into the right atrium via the superior vena cava (SVC) and the inferior vena cava (IVC). Then it enters the right ventricle (RV), and the pulmonary artery (PA) takes it to the lungs. Here, the blood gets oxygenated and returns to the left side of the heart through pulmonary veins.

This fresh blood gets into the left atrium (LA), left ventricle (LV), and is ejected again into the aorta (Ao) and the general arterial circulation.

THE VALVES

There are four cardiac valves. They are constantly opening and closing, opening and closing. The valves ensure that the blood moves in one direction only. Once they close tight, the valves prevent backflow. Blood is not allowed to leak back or regurgitate. A minimal amount of regurgitation is a normal occurrence in one or all the cardiac valves. It is called physiological regurgitation, and it is a normal event.

A moderate or severe leaking of any cardiac valve requires evaluation.

After blood returning from the body fills the right atrium, it is forced from the right atrium through the *tricuspid valve* into the right ventricle. The right ventricle pumps it through the *pulmonary valve* into the lungs.

At the same time that blood from the right atrium moves into the right ventricle, the blood returning from the lungs flows into the left atrium and passes through the *mitral valve,* reaching the left ventricle. Just as the right ventricle pumps blood to the lungs through the *pulmonic valve*, the left ventricle ejects blood into the aorta through the *aortic valve*.

THE MYOCARDIUM OR HEART MUSCLE

The muscular tissue that represents the heart pump is called *myocardium*. All four cardiac chambers—the left and right atria and left and right ventricles—are surrounded by myocardium. And the myocardium is covered by the *pericardium*. This is a double membrane that contains a small amount of fluid that acts as a lubricant.

THE CONDUCTING OR ELECTRICAL SYSTEM

The myocardium contracts when stimulated by an electrical current. The electricity that stimulates the heart originates in a tiny structure called the *sinoatrial node*, located at the right atrium. From here, the electrical current spreads through the atria and ventricles using a *conducting or wiring system*.

It is the *electrical stimulation* of the heart muscle or myocardium that produces the *mechanical stimulation* (contraction).

The heart is no ordinary pump. It has about the size of your fist, and in a period of seventy-five years, it contracts 3.26 billion times and ejects 57.5 million gallons of blood.

How many pumps do you know that are able to work so well for so long?

Figure 4. The Heart's Electrical System

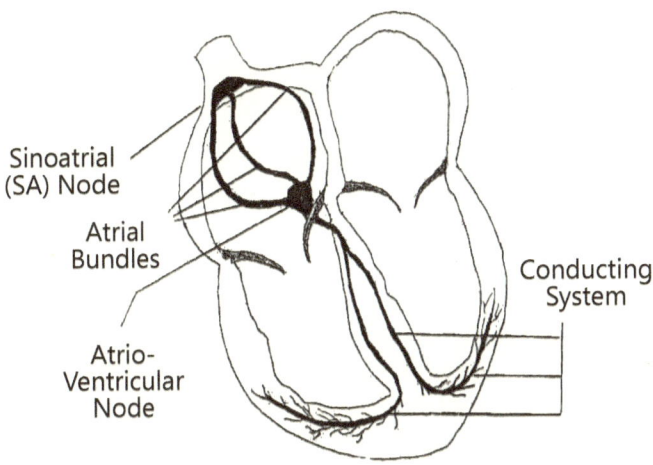

Sinoatrial
(SA) Node

Atrial
Bundles

Atrio-
Ventricular
Node

Conducting
System

THE CORONARY ARTERIES

These arteries originate from the aorta and provide blood to the heart muscle. The name "coronary" comes from "corona" that means "crown." They surround the heart like a crown. The right coronary artery supplies blood to the bottom and right side of the heart.

The left coronary arteries, which consist of two main branches, supply the rest.

Figure 5. The Coronary Arteries

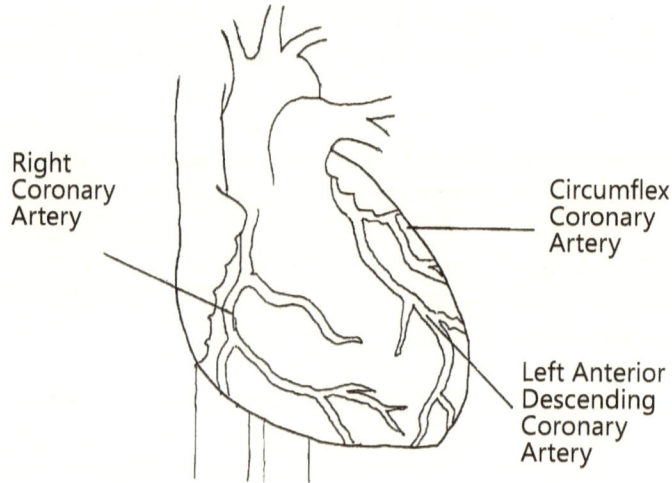

Right Coronary Artery

Circumflex Coronary Artery

Left Anterior Descending Coronary Artery

HOW DOES OBESITY DAMAGE THE HEART?

It does it through different mechanisms. It may damage the coronary arteries, the heart muscle, the conducting system, the valves, or any of the above in combination.

The heavier the weight, the more serious are the consequences.

CARDIAC ABNORMALITIES CAUSED BY OBESITY

- **Congestive heart failure**
    * Fluid overload
    * Fatty infiltration of cardiac tissue
    * Coronary atherosclerosis
    * Diabetes
    * Hypertension

- **Atrial fibrillation**
- **Malignant cardiac arrhythmias and sudden death**
- **Coronary artery disease: angina—myocardial infarction**
- **Hypertensive cardiovascular disease**

This chapter's explanations are a bit technical, but it's necessary to know how and why the circulatory system gets into trouble because of morbid obesity.

CONGESTIVE HEART FAILURE (CHF) IN THE OBESE PATIENT

CHF means that the heart is unable to provide the needed blood supply to various organs. In other words, the heart muscle, "the pump," is weak. If you lift and hold an object for a while, you'll experience fatigue. When the heart is forced to deal with a heavy burden, it bravely resists, but only for some time. When it can't take it anymore, it gives up.

In boxing terminology, the heart "throws the towel." In medical terminology, the condition is called *heart failure*: the heart loses its capacity to eject blood effectively into the circulation. This results in fluid accumulation—also called congestion—in the lungs, liver, and legs, resulting in shortness of breath (lung congestion), right upper abdominal discomfort and liver enlargement (liver congestion) and lower extremities edema (legs congestion). That is why the condition is called *congestive heart failure*.

CONGESTIVE HEART FAILURE IN OBESITY DUE TO FLUID OVERLOAD

The human body has two main compartments: (1) intravascular compartment (veins and arteries), and (2) extravascular compartment (tissues that surround veins and arteries).

Blood contained inside arteries and veins represents the *blood volume*. When there's blood loss—hemorrhage, gastrointestinal bleeding—the blood volume decreases. In other conditions, such as morbid obesity, *the blood volume increases*. Why? Because increased amount of fatty tissue demands a proportional increase in blood supply. This is done by an increase in blood volume, which occurs because fluid is *mobilized from the extravascular space into the vascular space*. This results in *circulatory overload*.

For a while ("a while" may be years), the heart function is not affected. Give it enough time, and there will be untoward consequences, such as a weakened heart muscle.

Figure 6. Increased fluid load gets into the circulation.

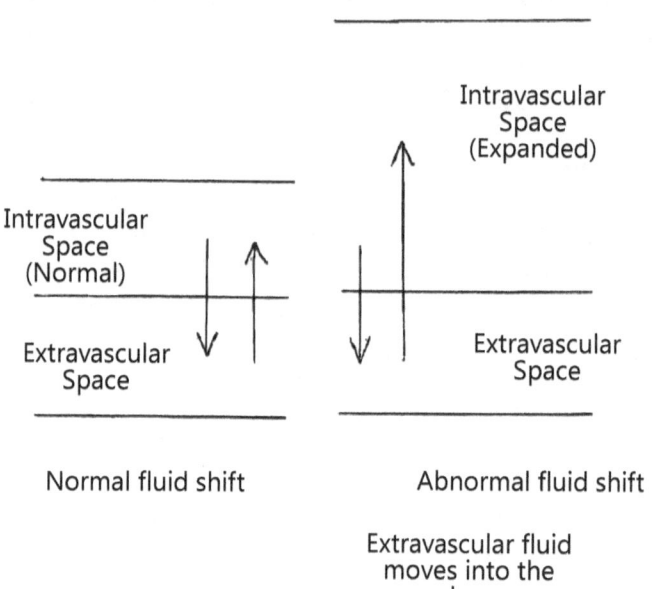

Normal fluid shift   Abnormal fluid shift

Extravascular fluid
moves into the
vascular space

The heart normally produces an average of eighty beats per minute (normal heartbeat is between sixty and one hundred beats per minute). *This equals to approximately 207 ½ million heartbeats in a five-year period.*

STROKE VOLUME AND CARDIAC OUTPUT

The amount of blood propelled into the general arterial system by the main heart pump, the left ventricle, *per beat*, is called *stroke volume*. The total amount of blood ejected by the left ventricle *per minute* is called *cardiac output*.

SEQUENCE OF EVENTS LEADING TO HEART FAILURE

When the blood volume expands as it happens in morbid obesity, there's an increased return of venous blood to the heart. This stretches the cardiac chambers. The enlargement of the left ventricular cavity is called *left ventricular dilation*. Eventually, other cardiac chambers will do the same. Stretching of the left ventricular walls causes *wall stress*. (Try prolonged stretching of your arm, and you'll notice the discomfort.) *The ventricle deals with this extra effort by exercising its muscle. Any muscle that exercises gets thicker. The heart muscle is no exception.* Any muscle, regardless of how powerful and thick it is, gives up when forced to work hard for a longer period than it's able to handle. The increased heart muscle thickness is called *left ventricular hypertrophy*. The weakness of the heart muscle is called *congestive heart failure*.

Figure 7. Normal Heart Wall Thickness

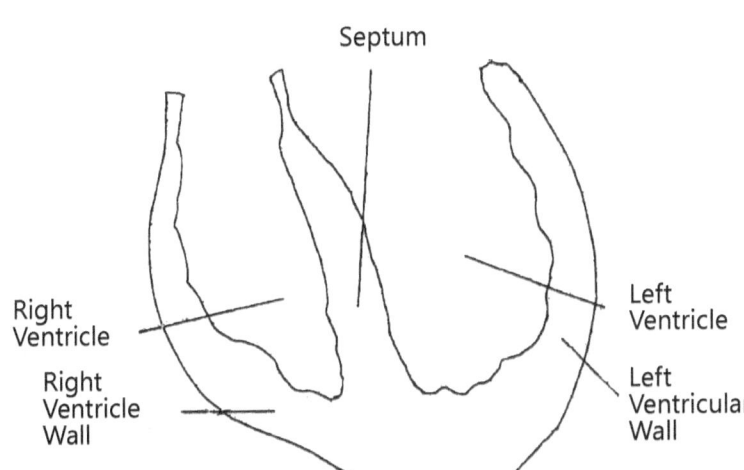

Figure 8. Thick Left Ventricle (Left Ventricular Hypertrophy)

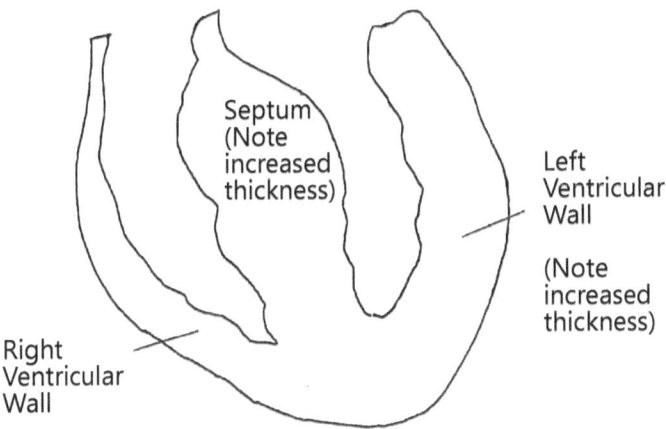

Figure 9. Dilated and Weakened Left Ventricle

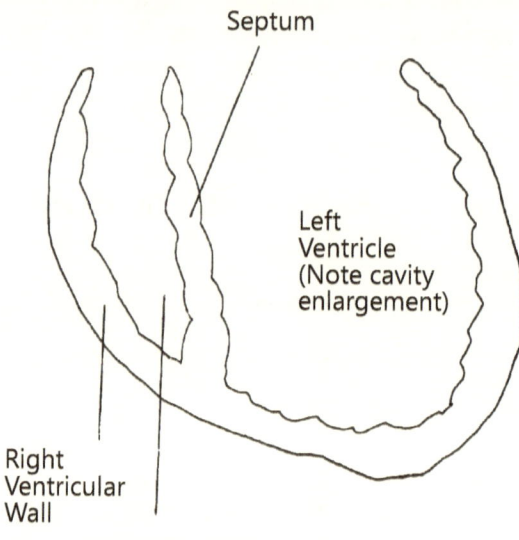

WHAT'S THE EJECTION FRACTION AND WHAT IT MEANS
====

Normally, when the left ventricle contracts and ejects blood into the circulation, it never empties 100 percent of the blood it contains. It ejects 50-75 percent of it. This is called the *ejection fraction*.

Ejection fraction (EF) is a very popular concept among cardiologists. There are different ways of knowing a person's ejection fraction. The most accessible and frequently used is the echocardiogram.

Then, if the left ventricle ejects 58 percent of its blood content, it means that its EF is 58 percent. In fact, any number between 50 percent and 75 percent is normal. A lower-than-normal EF indicates weakness of the heart muscle. Because the ejection of blood by the left ventricle with each heartbeat is called *systole, the ejection fraction is a measure of the left ventricular systolic function.*

Ejection Fraction

50-75 percent	=	**normal left ventricular systolic function**
40-49 percent	=	**mild impairment of left ventricular systolic function**

30-39 percent   =   **moderately severe impairment of left ventricular systolic function**

20-29 percent   =   **severe impairment of left ventricular systolic function**

19 percent or under   =   **very severe impairment of left ventricular systolic function**

To review:

1. **Obesity increases the demand for blood supply.** Reason: more fat needs more blood supply. (A bigger machine needs more fuel.)
2. **Circulating blood volume increases to satisfy that demand.** Mechanism: fluid moves from the extravascular space into the circulatory system.
3. **Increased blood volume means increased return of blood to the heart** through the venous system.
4. **Increased blood return to the heart results in dilation of the cardiac chambers.**
5. **Dilation of the left ventricle increases the stretching of its wall.** This means increased stress on those walls.
6. **Increased stress on the left ventricular walls means that the ventricle is forced to work harder.**
7. **Harder work leads to a thick left ventricular muscle**. This is called *left ventricular hypertrophy.*
8. **When the left ventricle (LV) gets tired of working hard, its contraction weakens, it is unable to empty itself appropriately, and the blood that stays behind accumulates in the lungs and other organs.** That is *heart failure.*

Symptoms of congestive heart failure include shortness of breath (due to fluid accumulation in the lungs' air spaces), coughing while lying flat (the body's horizontal position increases lung congestion, and that causes lung irritation and cough), nausea and abdominal discomfort located at the right upper quadrant of the abdomen due to liver congestion (increased amount of blood it contains), and edema of both lower extremities (swelling of legs and feet due to excessive fluid retention).

OBESITY

Increased Blood Volume

Increased Blood Return to the Heart

Heart Chambers Dilation

Stretching of the Left Ventricle Walls

Increased Left Ventricular Walls Stress

Harder Left Ventricle Work

Thick Left Ventricular Muscle
(LVH or Left Ventricular Hypertrophy)

If the above conditions persist,

CONGESTIVE HEART FAILURE

*   *   *

FATTY INFILTRATION OF THE HEART CAUSING HEART FAILURE

Cardiomyopathy of Obesity (*Adipositas Cordis*)

This condition is usually found in subjects who had severe and long-standing obesity. Adipose tissue covers the surface of the heart (*epicardium*), and *from here, cords of fat cells infiltrate the spaces in between the myocardial cells, exerting pressure on them, which leads to their atrophy.*

The cardiac cells are called *myocytes*. The coordinated action of the normal myocytes causes the normal cardiac contraction. The process that leads to inactivation of myocytes is called myocyte *degeneration. Loss of myocytes reduces the heart's contractile power.* The heart becomes flabby and weak (*congestive heart failure*).

Figure 10. Fatty Infiltration of the Myocardium (Heart Muscle)

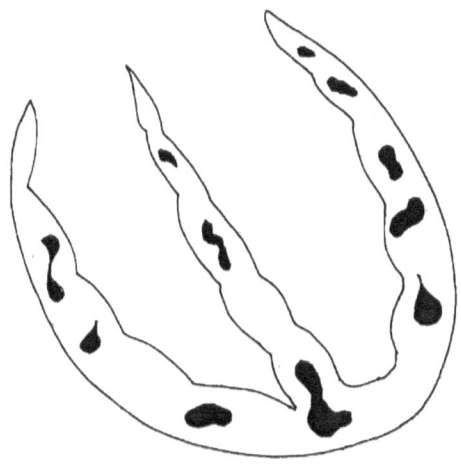

CONGESTIVE HEART FAILURE AND CORONARY ATHEROSCLEROSIS

Blockages of coronary arteries may lead to heart failure by causing

- severe chronic obstructions by atherosclerotic plaques (ischemic cardiomyopathy);
- extensive acute myocardial infarction;
- scar tissue left by an extensive myocardial infarction that produced a left ventricular aneurysm;
- acute complications of a myocardial infarction: heart perforation, ruptured papillary muscle, serious arrhythmias.

CONGESTIVE HEART FAILURE, OBESITY, AND DIABETES

Diabetics have a fivefold increased risk of developing heart failure.

Diabetes causes dysfunction of the cardiac cells (myocytes), and this leads to the so-called *diabetic cardiomyopathy* and heart failure.

The worse the diabetes status, the more significant the heart muscle damage.

Diabetes may also cause chest pains (angina) and congestive heart failure because of *microvascular dysfunction*. What is this?

Microvascular dysfunction means that the smallest branches of the coronary arteries—which are not visualized in the coronary angiogram—either constrict or fail to dilate when the heart muscle demands an increase in blood flow. The condition is called *microangiopathy* (from *micro* = "very small"; *angio* = "vessel"; *pathos* = "disease").

These changes in the heart muscle *"microcirculation"* may be associated with chest pains and abnormal ECG, but the *coronary angiogram may report "normal coronary arteries." The angiogram is able to detect abnormalities of the "major" coronary arteries, but abnormalities in the tiny branches evade angiographic recognition.*

Congestive heart failure in the diabetic patient may additionally result from either multiple coronary atherosclerotic obstructions or when one major coronary artery becomes blocked and causes an acute and severe myocardial infarction.

CONGESTIVE HEART FAILURE, SEVERE OBESITY, AND HYPERTENSION

Hypertension in the arterial system offers a resistance to the ejection of blood by the left ventricle into the circulation. In other words, the pump of the heart tries to push through blood, facing a higher-than-normal pressure in the arterial system. This means that the left ventricular muscle is overburdened. At one point, it gets fatigued (heart failure); the left ventricular cavity becomes dilated and flabby. This is called *hypertensive dilated cardiomyopathy.*

The frequent coexistence of coronary atherosclerosis, diabetes, and hypertension compounds the problem and facilitates the development of heart failure.

ATRIAL FIBRILLATION

This is a frequent rhythm disturbance that is more prevalent in obese persons. It is a *disorganized contraction of the atrial chambers* that produce a shivering-like motion in contrast with one single contraction per heartbeat that occurs in the normal heart.

The development of atrial fibrillation in the morbidly obese appears to be related to dilatation of the left atrial chamber. The stretching of the atrial muscle fibers alters the normal cardiac rhythm, which is replaced by multiple minicontractions of the atrial walls (atrial fibrillation).

When the arrhythmia is recurrent and alternates with periods of normal cardiac rhythm, it is called paroxysmal atrial fibrillation. If it becomes established and permanent, it is called chronic atrial fibrillation.

The frequent recurrence of the arrhythmia or its permanent presence may lead to complications: a fibrillating atrium delays the exit of blood from the atrium to the ventricle. That sluggishness tends to promote clot formation. If the clot is released, it moves into the left ventricle, and from here is ejected into the general circulation. If it lands in the brain, it causes a stroke. If it stops in the spleen, it causes acute left upper quadrant abdominal pain. If it goes down a leg artery, it blocks it. The leg and foot will be cold, bluish, pale, and painful.

The clot released from the left ventricle is called *embolus*. Because it enters the circulatory system, the process is called *systemic embolization*.

Figure 11. Normal Cardiac Rhythm

P wave (reflects atrial activity)   QRS complex (reflects ventricular activity)

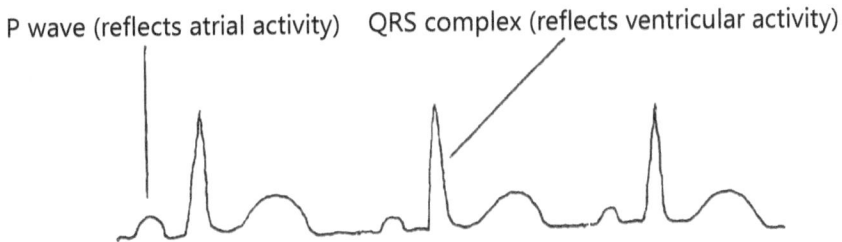

The normal process of electrical stimulation of the atria is expressed in the electrocardiogram by the P-wave. The stimulation of the ventricles shows a QRS complex. (Please see above.)

One atrial contraction leads to one ventricular contraction. Note the regularity of the rhythm. This is called sinus rhythm because it originates in an area located in the right atrium called the sinus node. From there, it spreads down to the rest of the heart using the conducting or cardiac electrical system.

Figure 12. Atrial Fibrillation

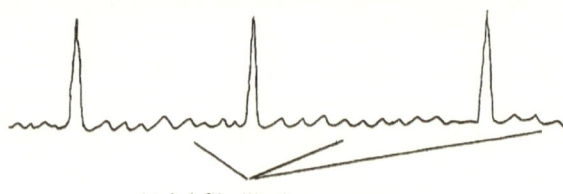

Atrial fibrillation waves

Note the absence of normal P-waves, which have been replaced by multiple waves that cause the shivering of the atrial chambers. One of these fibrillatory waves gets through the atrioventricular junction, and the ventricles become stimulated. This ventricular stimulation is irregularly spaced and so are the QRS complexes and the heartbeats that result from this abnormal cardiac activity.

MALIGNANT ARRHYTHMIAS AND SUDDEN DEATH

Obese patients, even those who are stable and have no objective evidence of cardiac dysfunction, may develop fatty tissue infiltration of the electrical wiring system of the heart, and this is associated with cardiac rhythm abnormalities: fast rhythms (tachycardia), slow rhythms (bradycardia).

Some of these arrhythmias are benign and cause no immediate trouble. Others are significant and may lead to fainting, palpitations, shortness of breath, chest pains, strokes, heart failure, or sudden death.

The Framingham study estimated that the annual incidence of sudden cardiac mortality rate in obese men and women was about forty times higher than the rate of unexplained cardiac arrest in a nonobese population.

Stable-weight obese individuals have an increased risk of sudden death even in the absence of cardiac dysfunction. In the specific case of severely obese men, a sixfold to twelvefold excess mortality rate has been reported.

Figure 13. Ventricular Tachycardia

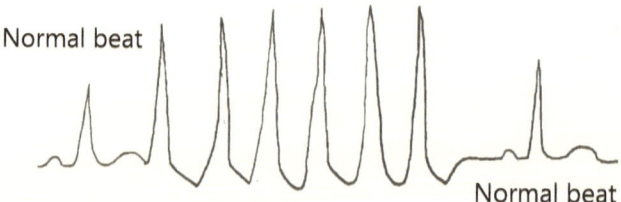

Normal beat

Normal beat

If uncorrected, it leads to ventricular fibrillation.

Figure 14. Ventricular Fibrillation

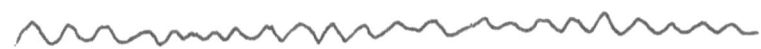

If uncorrected, it leads to total absence of electrical activity.

Figure 15. Cardiac Standstill
No electrical activity—the heart no longer contracts

(unless the situation is reversed by cardiopulmonary resuscitation).

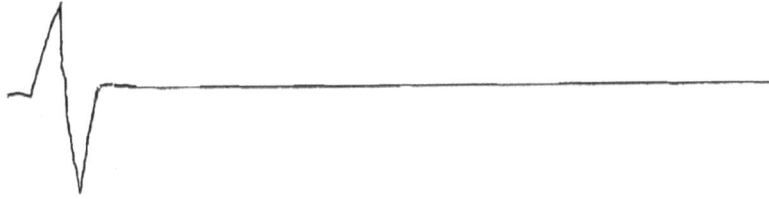

THE QT INTERVAL

A normal electrocardiogram shows the electrical activity of the atrial chambers (P-wave) and that of the ventricles (QT interval).

A significant percentage of obese persons have been found to have prolonged QT intervals and this is particularly so in the severely obese. This is important because prolonged QT intervals are known to be a risk factor for dangerous ventricular arrhythmias and sudden death.

Figure 16. A. Normal QT interval   B. Prolonged QT interval

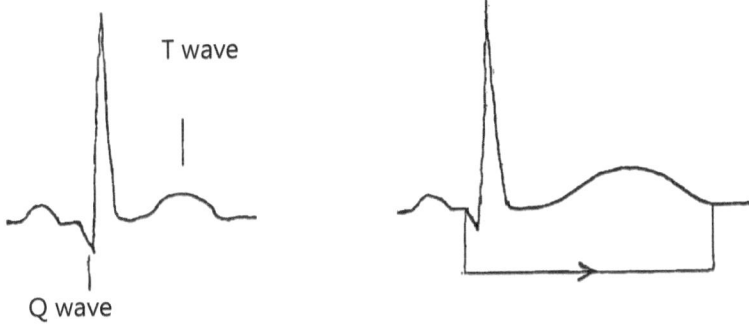

T wave

Q wave

CORONARY ARTERY DISEASE

(For additional information about atherosclerosis, please see chapter 3.)

Atherosclerotic plaques inside the coronary arteries often develop over a period of decades, frequently beginning during childhood as fatty deposits, called *fatty streaks*, and then slowly grow and become thicker due to the accumulation of calcium and other substances (atherosclerotic plaques) to the point where they partially or totally block the coronary artery causing chest pain or discomfort called angina pectoris and/or a myocardial infarction. Quite often, they are silent.

There are millions of individuals who have plaques of different shapes and sizes inside their coronary arteries and are totally unaware about their existence. (You probably had lunch with one of them today!)

These plaques *do not need to obstruct a coronary artery significantly to cause trouble. Soft and nonobstructive plaques* (nonobstructive plaques are those that do not block more than 50 percent of the artery) *can crack more easily because of their softness.*

When the plaque cracks, circulating blood components immediately form a clot. If it is small, it may not have significant consequences, particularly when the patient's own clot dissolving mechanisms dissolve it fast. If it's a large one, the coronary artery gets blocked, and an acute myocardial infarction develops.

So it is very important to understand that all coronary plaques are a potential source of trouble. Hard, severely obstructed plaques may cause an acute myocardial infarction because the blood does not get through the narrowed area of the artery.

Soft, nonobstructive plaques that block the artery less than 50 percent do not limit the blood supply to the heart muscle but must be watched for two reasons:

Reason no. 1. They may progress in size and increase the degree of blockage in the future.

Reason no. 2. Because these plaques are generally soft, they may crack more easily. Once this happens, a clot is form in that wounded area of the arterial wall, and if this is big enough, it may occlude the vessel completely. This results in an acute myocardial infarction.

Figure 17. Soft, fissured, nonobstructive plaque and clot formation

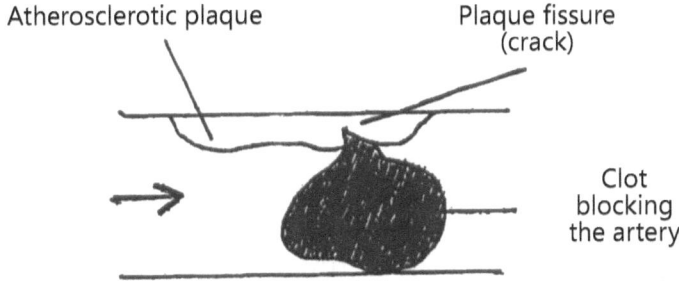

Atherosclerotic plaque

Plaque fissure (crack)

Clot blocking the artery

Figure 18. Hard, obstructive atherosclerotic plaque

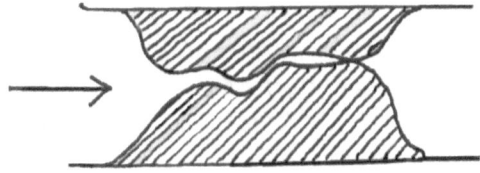

Figure 19. Myocardial infarction

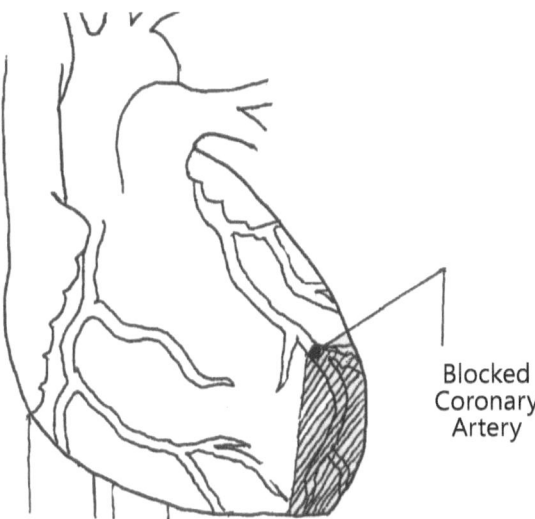

Blocked Coronary Artery

Two reputable studies, the Framingham Heart Study and the Manitoba Study, after a follow-up of twenty-six years, documented that obesity represents an independent predictor of cardiovascular disease, particularly in women. The association is stronger in people younger than fifty, reinforcing the concept that obesity leads to premature atherosclerosis.

A high BMI is significantly associated with myocardial infarction and sudden death.

When we say that obesity is associated with advanced atherosclerosis (which is true), we do not mean to say that *all* obese individuals are at high risk of cardiovascular disease. Those who carry other cardiovascular risk factors, such as high cholesterol and triglycerides blood levels or apolipoprotein B, fibrinogen high blood levels and/or other proclotting factors or have elevated blood levels of C-reactive protein are particularly susceptible for the development of coronary artery disease.

Distribution of body fat matters too. An abdominal preponderance is not only associated with increased incidence of coronary artery disease: an accelerated progression of carotid atherosclerosis has also been observed in men.

HYPERTENSIVE CARDIOVASCULAR DISEASE

Hypertension *is a treacherous condition. It may exist for decades without causing symptoms until a complication occurs.*

The damage caused in the cardiovascular system that results from hypertension is called *hypertensive cardiovascular disease.* This includes myocardial infarctions, congestive heart failure, cardiac rhythm disturbances, strokes, kidney failure, arteriosclerosis throughout the body, sexual dysfunction, retinal hemorrhages, and sudden death.

Morbid obesity and hypertension frequently coexist, and *a normal weight is an important component of any antihypertensive therapy.*

WHAT DOES IT TAKE TO SUCCEED?

- A desire to learn
- The process of learning
- The implementation of what you learned

- The willpower and consistency to comply with medical instructions on permanent basis

Morbid obesity is a dangerous condition that becomes even more so when the patient doesn't have the basic knowledge to deal with it.

Many tragedies could be prevented by acting rationally and effectively, making the right decisions at the right time.

If you are suffering from morbid obesity, you're running a race between future medical complications and your willingness and ability to avoid them.

Do whatever is in your power to be the winner.

CHAPTER 3

MORBID OBESITY, VASCULAR DISEASE, AND CLOTS: AWARENESS HELPS PREVENTION

Those who work underground often go undetected.

Cardiovascular risk factors are a potential source of trouble. Sometimes, big-time trouble! They act like conspirators, playing the role of undercover agents assigned to a deadly mission. Diabetes, hypertension, abnormal serum lipids levels, poor eating habits, stress, insufficient physical activity, unlucky genes that transmit the propensity to develop heart disease perform their misdeeds for long periods of times, usually decades, and during the process, they remain alarmingly silent until the day a cardiovascular complication comes into your life without asking you permission to do so.

In the preceding chapter, I described the behavior of atherosclerotic plaques inside the coronary arteries. Those plaques exist in arteries in different areas of the human anatomy. In this section, we'll briefly discuss how atherosclerosis affects the carotid-cerebral circulation, the aorta, the arteries that supply blood to abdominal organs and the lower extremities.

CEREBROVASCULAR DISEASE

The blood supply to the brain can be compromised temporarily or permanently. A temporary (transient) deficiency of blood supply means a process that lasts minutes to hours. It is defined as *TIA* (transient ischemic attack). *Ischemic* means "diminished blood supply." TIA typical examples are transient visual deficit, speech slurring, weakness of an arm or leg, episodes of confusion, and disorientation.

This may occur because of a little clot that travels from the left atrium or left ventricle to the brain or a partial obstruction of a carotid or cerebral artery.

When a traveling clot lodges in a cerebral artery and occludes it completely or the carotid artery is severely narrowed or a cerebral artery is totally occluded, a portion of the brain becomes damaged due to lack of blood supply. This is called a *stroke*. Because the affected area is deprived of blood, it is called *ischemic stroke*. The resulting damaged area of the brain is called *cerebral infarction*.

Figure 20. Carotid artery blockage

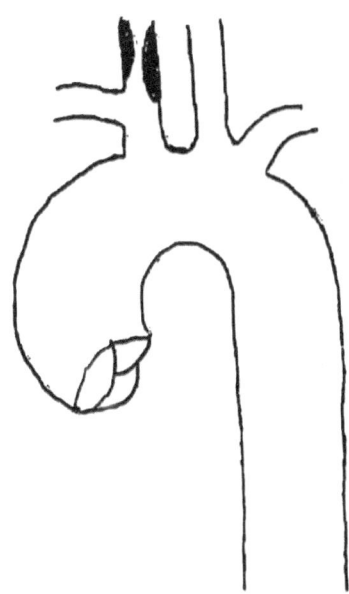

Figure 21. Ischemic stroke—Cerebral infarction Cerebral artery blockage

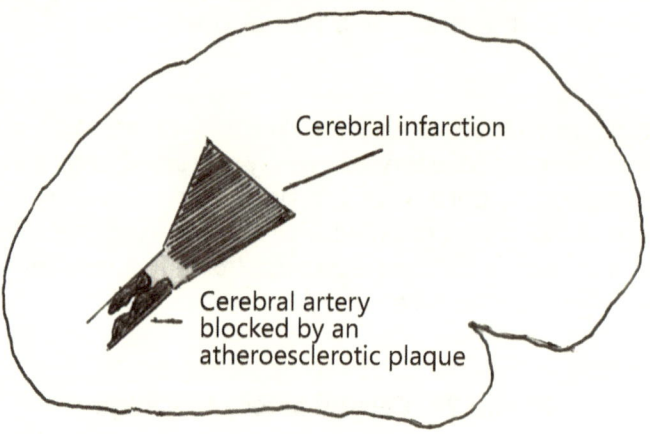

Cerebral infarction

Cerebral artery blocked by an atheroesclerotic plaque

Figure 22. Hemorrhagic stroke—Cerebral hemorrhage Rupture of a cerebral artery

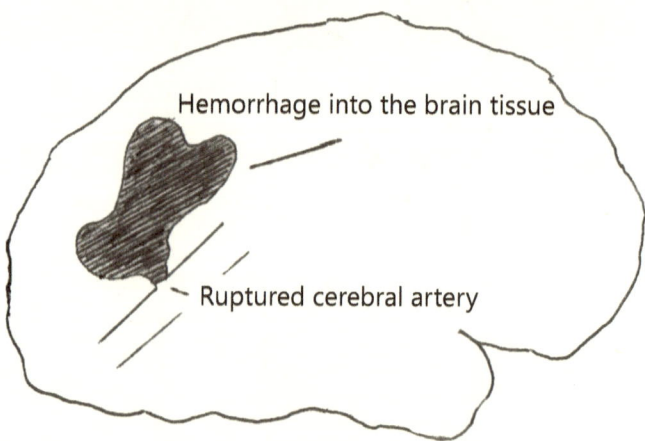

Hemorrhage into the brain tissue

Ruptured cerebral artery

**Some of the possible sites for clot formation
capable of traveling to the brain**

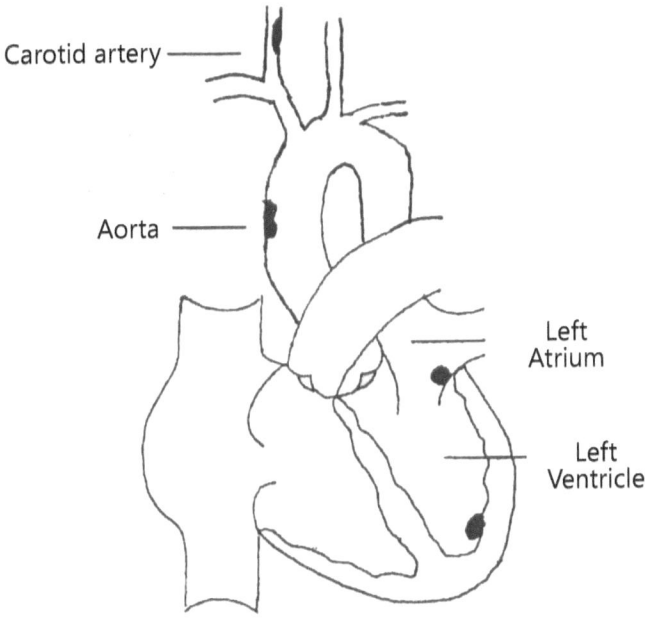

Carotid artery

Aorta

Left
Atrium

Left
Ventricle

When a cerebral artery bursts instead of being blocked, blood drains into the brain, and this is called hemorrhagic stroke or cerebral hemorrhage.

THORACIC AND ABDOMINAL AORTIC ANEURYSMS

Sometimes, atherosclerosis, by damaging the arterial wall, leads to abnormal, localized widening of the aorta called aneurysms. They are a great concern particularly when they involve the thoracic or abdominal aorta.

These mostly occur in long-standing hypertensive patients. Smoking is an important contributing factor. Obesity is frequently associated with hypertension. Aneurysms need close follow-up since they may increase in size without recognizable symptoms.

Aortic aneurysms may rupture. When they do, the patient's condition becomes critical.

An expanding thoracic aortic aneurysm may provide warning symptoms, such as shortness of breath, chest pain, pulsatile pain in the chest or head, pain in between the shoulder blades, hoarseness, and dry cough.

Abdominal aortic aneurysms in the obese can be very tricky due to the fact that a severely obese abdomen does not allow its detection by the palpating hand of the examiner.

Impending rupture of an abdominal aortic aneurysm may present with severe abdominal and low back pain but may also be disguised, and the patient just complains of mild, vague abdominal discomfort.

Ultrasound and CT scans establish the diagnosis. An acutely expanding aneurysm, regardless of its location, represents a medical-surgical emergency.

Figure 23.

A. Normal thoracic aorta   B. Thoracic aortic aneurysm

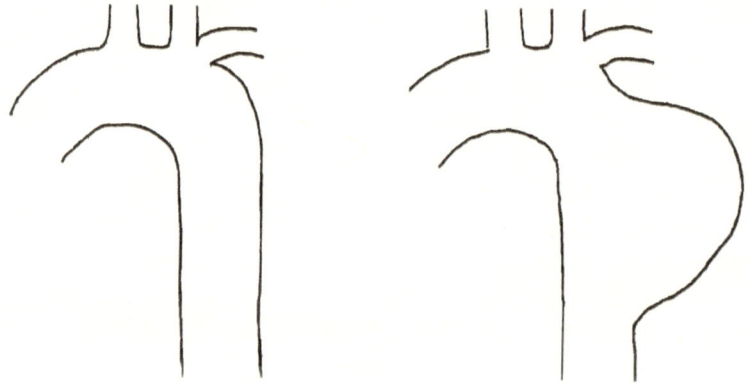

Figure 24.

A. Normal abdominal aorta B. Abdominal aortic aneurysm (AAA)

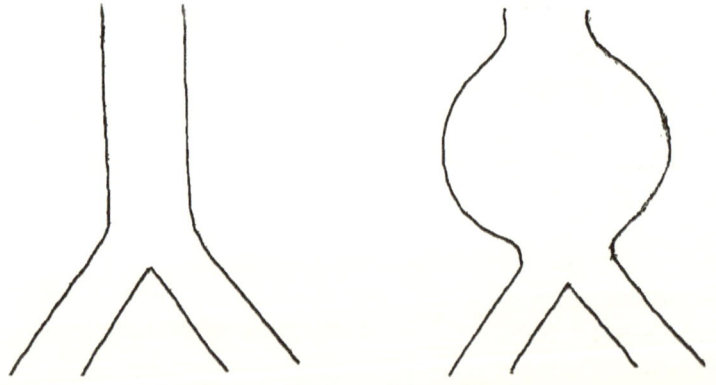

MESENTERIC ARTERY INSUFFICIENCY
(also called ABOMINAL ANGINA)

A blockage of the mesenteric artery (it supplies blood to the intestine) may cause abdominal pain following meals. It is known as abdominal angina or *ischemic bowel disease*.

RENAL ARTERY STENOSIS (RAS)

Stenosis is the medical term for "narrowing." RAS or renal artery stenosis is a severe blockage of a renal artery. The most frequent cause of renal artery blockage in the elderly is an atherosclerotic plaque. This deprives the kidney of adequate blood supply. The kidney reacts to this provocation by producing substances that constrict arteries throughout the body. That causes hypertension, usually of severe degree, and not very responsive to usual antihypertensive medications.

This kind of hypertension can be improved and even be cured by dilating the renal artery with a balloon and placing a stent to keep it open, like it is done in other areas of the body.

Figure 25. Blocked renal artery

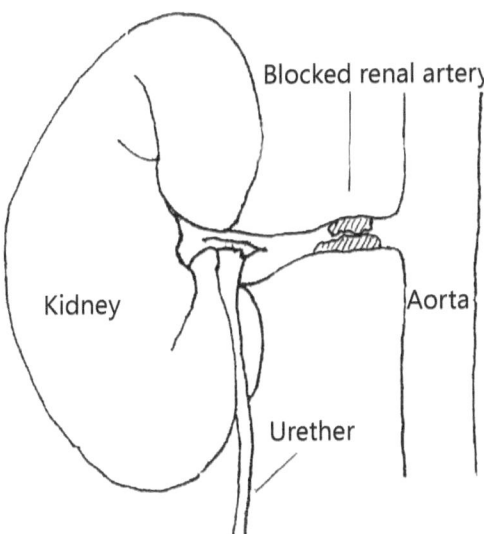

**Obstructed Renal Artery
by an atherosclerotic plaque**

ILIAC FEMORAL AND LOWER EXTREMITIES ARTERIES

These can be blocked due to the following:

Figure 26. Iliac artery blockage

A. Thick Atherosclerotic Plaques

B. Clots from the Left Atrium and Left Ventricle

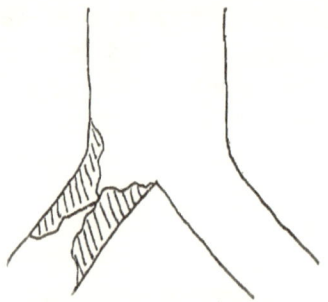   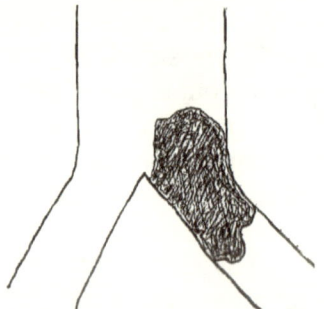

A- Atherosclerotic plaque   **B- Clot thrown by the heart**

Occlusion of the iliac femoral or lower extremities arteries can cause pain on walking, usually in the calf area, called intermittent claudication, in addition to foot complications, such as ulcers, infections, severe pain (due to deficient blood supply), or gangrene.

IMPOTENCE-ERECTILE FAILURE DUE TO BLOCKAGE OF THE PENILE ARTERIES

DISEASES OF THE VENOUS SYSTEM

Veins are conduits that carry blood back to the heart.

Damage to the inner layer of the wall of a vein stimulates clotting substances of the circulating blood to form a clot called thrombus. The process is called thrombosis.

Veins have valves. Incompetence of these valves leads to reflux of blood (venous insufficiency). Normally, blood is carried by the veins toward the heart and veins valves close and prevent reflux of blood. When veins and their valves become weak and insufficient, the valves do not close properly and allow the regurgitation of blood that moves in an opposite direction. It moves backward, back to the legs and feet.

That excess of blood in the lower extremities increases the venous pressure, and this dilates the veins producing varicosities. This raised pressure inside the veins pushes fluid out of them, and this accumulates in the surrounding tissues. That fluid accumulation is called edema.

Chronic significant reflux of blood into superficial veins causes local skin changes, such as brownish pigmentation, and in more severe cases, ulcerations.

The formation of blood clots inside the deep veins is called DVT (deep venous thrombosis).

Obesity is associated with immobility. This leads to reduced velocity of venous flow (stasis), local damage of the vein wall, and increased tendency for clot formation.

A venous clot (thrombus) may remain attached to the vein wall or turn lose and travel to the lung (pulmonary embolus).

The detection of DVT (deep venous thrombosis) by physical examination is difficult. It is missed 50 percent of the time. Diagnostic testing must be done to improve the accuracy of the diagnosis. Doppler ultrasound has become the mainstay examination to detect or exclude DVT although this technique is not totally accurate either. Clinical judgment must be exercised by the health care practitioner in doubtful cases.

When DVT is diagnosed or seriously suspected, the patient must be treated with blood thinners—anticoagulants—to avoid propagation of the clot and its release into the venous circulation that means a certain destination to the lung.

A small pulmonary embolus can be treated medically, and the patient is expected to recover. A large clot that blocks a major branch of the pulmonary artery means real trouble (please see below).

Figure 27.

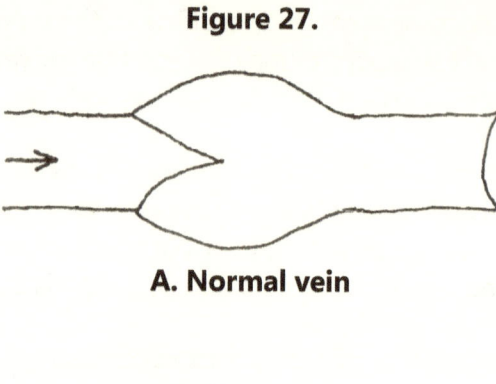

A. Normal vein

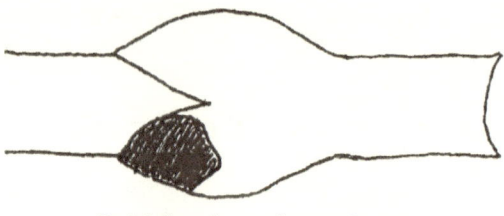

B. Vein clot (thrombus)

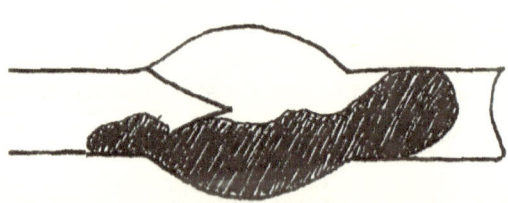

C. Propagation of a thrombus

PREVENTIVE MEASURES TO REDUCE THE RISK OF DVT IN PATIENTS WHO UNDERGO BARIATRIC SURGERY

Obese patients are at increased risk of venous clot formation in lower extremities, and after bariatric surgery, this is a great concern.

What is done to prevent DVT (deep venous thrombosis)

- Early postoperative ambulation
- Use of lower extremities compression devices
- Unless there's a contraindication for their use, these patients are given anticoagulants

Contraindications for the use of anticoagulants:
- Known allergy to the anticoagulant
- Heparin-induced thrombocytopenia (low platelet count)
- Blood coagulation disorder
- Active bleeding
- High risk of bleeding

NOTE

- The choice of the anticoagulant and duration of treatment needs to be individualized.
- When a venous clot is thought to represent a high risk for pulmonary embolization, an inferior vena cava filter needs to be considered.
- The most efficient implementation of clots preventive measures reduce but do not completely eliminate the possibility of their formation.

OBESITY AND LYMPHEDEMA

The lymphatic system consists of a series of vessels that are spread throughout the human body and whose function is the transport and drainage of fluid from the tissues into the venous system.

Lymph circulates in between cells, collects the waste resulting from the blood nourishment of the tissues, and moves into the veins. This activity is disturbed by obesity. Adipose cells (fatty cells) increase in number and size. This generates more cellular activity and the need to remove those waste products. The excess fatty tissue overcomes the capacity of the lymph vessel to do their job and compresses them. This raises the pressure inside the lymphatic vessels that leads to the exit of fluid into the tissues, causing their swelling. This kind of edema is different than the edema caused by venous insufficiency: edema due to deficient lymphatic drainage is harder to palpation and does not leave a mark as visible as the edema due to venous insufficiency.

CLOTS

Traveling clots are as preoccupying as their target sites.

Clots can be lifesaving. When there's a bleeding process, the formation of a clot is a blessing. If the blood didn't clot, we would continue to bleed, and naturally, that's not good.

On the other hand, when a clot forms inside the heart or a vessel (an artery or a vein), it isn't what you'd particularly call a happy medical event. In fact, it's a problem. At this point, the main medical concern is to make sure that the clot stays where it is and will not be fired into the venous system or the arterial system, whatever the case might be.

The best solution for clots in the circulation is their prevention. Physicians and surgeons always think about clots. They constantly worry about them. They have to.

Clots may form inside the heart, an artery, or a vein.

Clots are prone to form in the left atrium when the patient has an arrhythmia called atrial fibrillation. The atrial chambers do not contract forcefully but weakly with multiple erratic, feeble waves. These cause sluggishness of the circulation inside the left atrium and a tendency to form clots. That's why patients with this arrhythmia are usually treated with blood thinners (anticoagulants).

After a severe myocardial infarction, sometimes the damaged area promotes clot formation in the affected area of the left ventricle. This is another place inside the heart where clots may be ready to get fired into the arterial system.

Clots that are released from the heart into the general circulation have an unpredictable itinerary. Because these clots are thrown into the circulatory system, the process is called *systemic embolization.* If a clot moves north and reaches the brain, a stroke results. If it goes south, it may reach the spleen, intestinal arterial vessels, the lower extremities, among other destinations. Symptoms depend upon the clot's landing site: If the spleen is involved, the patient will have acute pain in the left upper quadrant of the abdomen. If the intestinal artery is the recipient of the clot, the symptom will be diffuse abdominal pain. If the clot blocks an artery of the lower extremity, the leg and the foot will be pale and bluish or may show gangrene.

A clot released by the venous system, contrary to a clot released by the left atrium or left ventricle, *almost always* has a predictable itinerary. When it originates in a vein of the leg or thigh, it is carried by the blood of the inferior vena cava that drains it into the right side of the heart, and from there, it moves to the lung (*pulmonary embolization*).

But there's an exception. Occasionally, a clot released by a vein of the lower extremity may reach the right atrium and from here passes into the left atrium through a little hole in the interatrial septum (a piece of tissue that separates both atrial chambers). From the left atrium goes to left ventricle and the general arterial circulation. This condition is called *paradoxical embolization.*

A small pulmonary embolus causes some chest pain, tachycardia, and shortness of breath and may be resolved by natural defense mechanisms that dissolve the clot or appropriate medical therapy. A large pulmonary embolus that blocks a major branch of a pulmonary artery may be fatal.

The purpose of anticoagulation therapy is to

A. **avoid an increase in size of the clot,**
B. **avoid the formation of other clots,**
C. **avoid the release or dislodgement of the clot.**

To sum it up:

1. Morbid obesity is associated with atherosclerotic heart disease, hypertensive cardiovascular disease, congestive heart failure, heart attacks (myocardial infarctions), left atrial and left ventricular chambers dilatation, and atrial fibrillation, all of which predispose to clot formation inside the left atrium or ventricle from where the clots can be fired into the arterial circulatory system.
2. Morbid obesity is associated with venous disease of the lower extremities (varicosities and peripheral venous insufficiency)—poor drainage of blood from those veins—that leads to clot formation. When the clot is released, it travels to the lungs (pulmonary embolus).

To prevent formation or release of clots *from the cardiac chambers,* anticoagulants are used.

To prevent formation or release of clots *from the venous system,* anticoagulants are used *in addition to* increased motion of lower extremities, early postoperative ambulation, and elastic stockings. At times, a filter is placed in the inferior vena cava to prevent clots from reaching the lungs.

To reduce the formation and release of *all kinds of clots, cardiac, arterial, or venous clots, obesity must be either prevented or corrected.*

First things first. Don't you agree?

CHAPTER 4

THE RESPIRATORY TRACT AND MORBID OBESITY: SLEEP APNEA AND LUNG DISEASE

All morbidly obese patients have shortness of breath on moderate exertions. Ten percent of them have severe respiratory impairment.

Respiratory insufficiency of obesity consists of two main breathing disorders:

1. **The obstructive sleep apnea syndrome (OSAS) and**

2. **The obesity hypoventilation syndrome (OHS)**

The combination of 1 and 2 represents a particularly severe form of respiratory impairment, and it is called the Pickwickian syndrome, which is the association of obesity, excessive somnolence, and carbon dioxide retention.

The name Pickwickian originated from Charles Dickens's novel *Pickwick Papers*. A fat boy named Joe had all the classical symptoms of the disorder and went into history with this designation.

Weight loss markedly improves or corrects respiratory insufficiency secondary to obesity. The lungs expand much better, and this improves arterial oxygenation and minimizes CO_2 retention. (CO_2 retention is another sign of poor ventilation.)

Severe respiratory insufficiency associated with obesity demands an aggressive approach to weight reduction.

SLEEP APNEA: FROM NOISY BREATHING TO A DISTURBING SILENCE

It is easier to find something when you know what you are looking for.

Many patients will not tell the health care provider that they snore at night, and that they are sleepy during daytime. The professional must directly and specifically ask for symptoms that may result from sleep apnea.

During my interviews with patients, they seldom volunteer this information. When I question them on these symptoms, they quickly admit having them. *Sleep apnea is an underdiagnosed illness.*

These are the appropriate questions:

- **Do you have disturbed sleep at night?**
- **Do you snore during the sleep?**
- **Do you doze off more than you should or feel sleepy at daytime?**

Those who live alone may not know whether they snore or not.

A little snoring here and there during the sleep, *not associated with sleep disruption* (waking up every hour or two), may not be a serious problem. A deviated nasal septum can cause it.

Anyone who involuntarily stops breathing for longer than ten seconds is said to have suffered an episode of *apnea*. Morbidly obese patients often stop breathing while sleeping. This results from upper airway obstruction. The condition is called *obstructive sleep apnea (OSA)*.

Since their sleep is interrupted several times during the night because of choking spells, they suffer from daytime sleepiness. This, under certain circumstances, may have serious consequences: impaired work performance, e.g., security, air-traffic comptrollers, increased sick leave, higher divorce rate, increased risk for motor accidents.

CONTRIBUTING FACTORS FOR OBSTRUCTIVE SLEEP APNEA (OSA)

1. **Obesity** *is one of the most important risk factors for obstructive sleep apnea (OSA).* Narrowing of the upper airway is the result of *excessive fat deposits in the neck.* The size of the neck due to marked fat deposition is a good predictor of sleep apnea. Abdominal obesity has also been correlated with sleep apnea.
2. **Supine posture** reduces upper-airway size.
3. Obese persons who suffer from sleep apnea often have *larger tongue (macroglossia) and smaller upper airway than nonobese individuals.*
4. **Swelling of the upper airways** due to *edema produced by vibrations resulting from prolonged snoring* may be a significant contributor in some cases.
5. **Age.** OSA increases with age. This may be related to loss of elasticity in the upper airway tissues.
6. **Gender.** After menopause, there is decreased elasticity of the upper airway due to estrogen deficiency and this predisposes to OSA
7. **Genetics and maxillofacial abnormalities.** Independent of obesity, there is a familial incidence of OSA and deficient occlusion of the mandible.
8. **Large tonsils and adenoids**
9. **Abnormal high-arched palates**
10. **Nasal obstruction** due to polyps or deviated septum

Note: 7, 8, 9, and 10 may cause OSA in patients who are not obese.

In cases of severe obesity, the neck fatty tissue interferes with the action of normal neck muscles in charge of dilating the airway. Infiltration with adipose tissue weakens these muscles. Inadequate opening of the upper airway translates into airway obstruction. The situation gets worse during the sleep because the muscular tone and strength—both of which are responsible for opening up or dilating the airway—are reduced.

CHANGES IN BLOOD GASES CONCENTRATION

Normal respiratory function is expressed by normal concentration of oxygen and carbon dioxide in arterial blood. In morbid obesity, the concentration of oxygen in arterial blood is lower than normal. This is called *hypoxemia.* In some cases, there is concomitant elevation of carbon dioxide, and this is *hypercapnia.* The combination of hypoxemia and hypercapnia causes disruption of sleep. If severe, it can lead to a cardiac arrest.

SYMPTOMS OF SLEEP-TROUBLED BREATHING

* Snoring
* Daytime sleepiness. Falling asleep during driving has caused accidents. It may also impair work performance due to fatigue and loss of concentration.
* Sleep interruptions at night
* Gasping or choking during sleep
* Morning headaches
* Poor memory
* Deficient concentration
* Fatigue
* Sexual dysfunction (reduced libido and erectile failure)
* Irritability and moodiness

Some of the above are only noted by relatives or a bed partner.

HOW IS OBSTRUCTIVE SLEEP APNEA DIAGNOSED?

The best method is an overnight in-laboratory sleep study (polysomnography or *PSG*).

Breathing patterns are evaluated; samples of arterial oxygen and carbon dioxide concentration and oxygen saturation are obtained. The patient is also monitored during a full sleep by two electrode-encephalogram channels, eye-movement recording channels, and one electromyogram channel and measure of airflow at the nose and/or mouth.

In some instances, a patient who suffers from OSA may not show abnormalities during this testing. When there is significant suspicion about the diagnoses, the sleep study may need to be repeated.

PSG study is expensive and inconvenient. At times, one can be satisfied with the diagnosis of OSA when oxygen concentration in arterial blood samples fall during the night.

TREATMENT OF OBSTRUCTIVE SLEEP APNEA (OSA)

1. **Weight loss** by caloric restriction or bariatric surgery significantly decrease the severity of OSA.

2. **Watch out alcohol and tranquilizers.** These can reduce pharyngeal muscle tone and depress arousal responses. The combination of these two leads to longer periods of sleeping apnea.
3. **Smoking aggravates OSA** by causing airway inflammation.
4. **Supine position makes OSA worse,** and it should be avoided. A tennis ball apply to the back may help some patients to avoid that position.
5. **Any cause of nasal obstruction should be corrected.**
6. The **CPAP machine** delivers positive pressure through the mouth or nose thereby preventing closure of the airway. How much pressure is necessary? It varies from four to 20 centimeters of water. The main objection to the use of the CPAP machine is *compliance*, which is only between 40 and 70 percent.
7. **Mandibular advancement devices** (MADs) are intraoral orthodontic devices that displace the mandible anteriorly, thus increasing the diameter of the upper airway preventing its collapse. They should be worn during the night. Patients who can't tolerate the CPAP machine may benefit from a MAD.
8. **Surgery**
    *   **Tracheostomy.** This is an opening created in the trachea to allow airflow to the lungs when the OSA is so severe that the upper airways do not allow enough air passage. It is only used as a last resort.
    *   **Uvulopalatopharyngoplasty and other upper-airway surgery.** These involve uvula or soft palate resection with or without the tonsils' removal.

Treatment of sleep apnea may be lifesaving.

LUNG DISORDERS ASSOCIATED WITH MORBID OBESITY

OBESITY HYPOVENTILATION SYNDROME (OHS)

Normal ventilation means that the lungs will absorb an adequate amount of oxygen and eliminate an adequate amount of CO_2 (carbon dioxide). Hypoventilation means that the lungs will not absorb enough oxygen or will retain more CO_2 than they are supposed to, or a combination of both.

Obesity hypoventilation syndrome (OHS) is typically seen in very severely obese patients (over 350 pounds).

Fat deposition in the muscles of the thorax reduces their mechanical strength and the depth of inspiration. As a result, lung volumes are reduced. This translates into defective oxygen uptake by the lungs and, at times, excessive retention of CO_2. These are the components of the OHS.

Symptoms include episodes of drowsiness or falling asleep at the wrong time during waking hours (narcosis), which is caused by the buildup of toxic levels of CO_2 in the blood.

OTHER BREATHING PROBLEMS ASSOCIATED WITH MORBID OBESITY

Morbid obesity is frequently associated with other lung diseases, and not surprisingly, during those circumstances, the patient's breathing capacity and the general medical status deteriorate further. This occurs with the following:

- Acute myocardial infarction
- Acute pneumothorax (lung collapse)
- Asthma and bronchitis
- Cardiac arrhythmia
- Cardiomyopathy
- Chronic obstructive pulmonary disease (emphysema)
- Congestive heart failure
- Coronary insufficiency (angina pectoris)
- Hyperventilation due to anxiety or panic attack
- Pneumonia
- Poor physical conditioning
- Previous lung resection for cancer
- Pulmonary embolism
- Valvular heart disease

SLEEPINESS IN THE OBESE PATIENT

Morbid obesity is just one of the causes of sleepiness in the obese patient. Other possible causes should be excluded.

- Hypnotics
- Alcohol abuse
- Drug abuse
- Narcolepsy

- Idiopathic somnolence
- Insomnia
- Occupations such as shift work and night shift, commercial drivers

I hope this chapter contributed to your better understanding of the mechanisms that cause shortness of breath in morbid obesity. Your family doctor with the help of a cardiologist, lung specialist, and at times, ear, nose, and throat consultant will perform the required testing and will determine what sections of the respiratory system are compromised and what should be done to correct them.

CHAPTER 5

OBESITY SURGERY
SHOULD YOU HAVE IT OR NOT?

In difficult life situations, questions and answers constantly wrestle with each other, competing for the truth.

The following are the clinical guidelines for consideration of weight-loss surgery.

A person qualifies for weight-loss surgery if he or she

1. has a BMI of 40 or more or a BMI of 35 or more in association with one or more major obesity-related medical or physical conditions;
2. has failed all previous attempts at weight reduction by conventional, conservative, and traditional methods (diet, exercise, behavior modification);
3. has no history of alcohol or substance abuse or has been completely rehabilitated;
4. is fully aware of the risks associated with surgery and accepts them;
5. commits him or herself prior to surgery to a permanent dedication to achieve radical lifestyle changes, dietary restrictions, regular exercises, long-term follow-up by the surgeon or bariatrician, and attend support groups when necessary;
6. has realistic expectations of surgical outcome;
7. qualifies psychologically for the operation. This is determined by a preoperative psychological evaluation;
8. does not have any medical, surgical, psychological, or psychiatric disorders that contraindicate weight-loss surgery (WLS).

A medically-supervised weight-reduction program should be attempted before the surgical approach to the treatment of morbid obesity is entertained. This is important for the following reasons:

1. It is a practical demonstration by the patient that he or she is capable of following guidelines of food restrictions that will be needed after surgery.
2. Even a small amount of weight loss prior to surgery will contribute to the reduction in the incidence of operative complications.

ADDITIONAL ELIGIBILITY CONSIDERATIONS

Do you have the right character and personality to go through this process?

Are you ready to commit yourself to a lifelong, radically different way of eating, sacrifice foods you love, accept others you never ate previously, and exercise regularly?

Do you realize that foods you used to enjoy will give you nausea, vomiting, upper chest discomfort, choking sensation, and other unpleasant symptoms?

Do you clearly understand that successful bariatric surgery will convert you physically, psychologically, and emotionally into a different person?

Are you ready to accept or deal with reactions of "friends," acquaintances, first-degree relatives, second-degree relatives, third-degree relatives, husband, wife, fiancée, or sexual partner?

The treatment approach to morbid obesity by diet, exercise, medications (pharmacological therapy), and behavioral therapy is *generally* ineffective. The "cure" rate for morbid obesity, using nonsurgical methods, is less than 5 percent.

Gastric surgery for obesity produces an average weight loss of fifty-five to ninety-seven pounds (twenty-five to forty-four kilograms) after one to two years. Patients usually lose about 70 percent of their excess body weight in one to two years.

Weight-loss surgery can dramatically improve or normalize many of obesity comorbidities.

IMPORTANT FACTS ABOUT WLS

* It is not a cure for eating disorders, but it helps to control the disease.
* It is not cosmetic surgery. The overriding reason to have this kind of surgery should not be physical looks but living a healthier, longer, and happier life.
* It is major surgery and has the potential for serious complications, including disability and loss of life.
* WLS is not the solution for morbid obesity. It is *only* part of the solution.
* WLS is a major decision. It shouldn't be considered until less-dramatic approaches (diet, exercise, drugs in some cases) are undertaken.

WHEN BARIATRIC SURGERY SHOULD NOT BE DONE

Following is the list of psychological or physical reasons that *disqualify* a person for weight-loss surgery.

Some conditions that contraindicate bariatric surgery at one particular point may be corrected with appropriate treatment, and patients may become acceptable candidates for weight-loss surgery.

a. **Cardiac**
   Severe heart disease
   Recent myocardial infarction
   Unstable angina

b. **Medical**
   Serious neurological conditions
   Overactive or underactive thyroid
   Cancer treatment
   Some gastrointestinal disorders
   Recent major surgery

c. **Psychiatric or Psychological**
   Emotional instability
   Severe anxiety (*)
   Severe depression (*)
   Uncontrolled bulimia
   Uncontrolled binges
   History of anorexa nervosa
   Bipolar disorder (manic-depressive states) (*)

Schizophrenia (*)
Other mental or psychological disorders

(*) Properly compensated anxiety, depression, schizophrenia, and bipolar disorders may qualify for weight-loss surgery.

Psychiatric and psychological dysfunctions require careful individualized approach, and a psychotherapist consultation is essential prior to deciding for obesity surgery.

EXAMPLE OF A PSYCHOLOGICAL DYSFUNCTION AND MORBID OBESITY THAT WAS NOT SUPPOSED TO BE TREATED BY WLS, BUT IT WAS!

A thirty-eight-year-old female patient carried 180 pounds of weight excess and requested bariatric surgery. She was emotionally unstable and had severe chronic anxiety and binges attacks.

I thought her psychological problems disqualified her—at least at that moment—for any kind of weight-loss surgery, and instead, recommended a consultation with a psychotherapist. She rejected my recommendation and went to another state where she had gastric band and stapling surgery.

After an initial modest loss, she gained all her weight excess back, and more. She couldn't swallow comfortably many foods she was craving for, but she gave herself a green light to eat "gallons of ice cream." The ice cream melted quickly, and it easily got through her tiny stomach pouch.

Conclusion: She should have resolved her psychological dysfunctions first and then consider WLS. She did exactly the opposite. That sequence should never be expected to work.

I insist on this: bariatric surgery doesn't stand a chance to succeed unless the patient has the right attitude and capacity to radically modify his or her lifestyle with respect to dietary restrictions, regular exercise, and medical follow-up.

Finding who qualifies for obesity surgery is a search that explores the patient's character and personality, his/her mental status and medical condition, and analyzes data that will be used by professionals who want you to succeed, enjoy your life, and be as healthy and happy as anyone can possibly be.

CHAPTER 6

SURGICAL TREATMENT
OF MORBID OBESITY

Drastic changes in our lives are only one inch away from a major decision.

Obesity surgery has become increasingly more accepted and popular in the last few years.

The classical gastric bypass operation requires an incision that is made from the breastbone to the nable. The laparoscopic technique involves several puncture holes through which a miniature camera is inserted to guide the surgery.

During the period between 1998 and 2002, weight-loss surgeries in the United States increased 450 percent to more than seventy-two thousand in 2002. The number progressively increased, and in 2005, 129,000 operations were performed.

Over 90 percent of all the weight-loss surgical procedures involve the Roux-en-Y procedure.

The use of laparoscopic technique grew from 2 percent of all bariatric surgical procedures in 1998 to nearly 18 percent in 2002. And the numbers continue to increase. It is anticipated that the laparoscopic approach will become more common than open surgery due to the "expansion era" pioneered by Dr. Alan Wittgrove, who just, a few years ago introduced the laparoscopic approach.

And it makes sense. There is a difference on the size of the incision—a rather large one in the upper part of the abdomen for the classical operation versus a few barely visible little "holes" in the abdominal wall when the laparoscopic method is used—the length of hospitalization is reduced and so are some of the postoperative complications, such as the incidence of pulmonary emboli and wound infections, more frequently seen in patients who undergo the classical major abdominal incision.

Complications, though, may occur from both the open abdominal surgery and the laparoscopic approach, with a death rate of about 0.19 percent *in the best centers.*

Approximately, nine million people in the United States are morbidly obese.

There are different kinds of surgical procedures to deal with morbid obesity. Which one is the best? The patient must discuss this issue with the surgeon.

There are pros and cons for every particular situation and what is the best method for one person may not be the appropriate option for another.

Currently, there are five major types of obesity surgery: the vertical banded gastroplasty (VBG), the adjustable gastric band (AGB), the sleeve gastrectomy (SG), the gastric bypass (GBP), also called the Roux-en-Y gastric bypass (RYGBP), and the biliopancreatic diversion with duodenal switch (BPD/DS).

Of all obesity surgical procedures, the Roux-en-Y gastric bypass is the most commonly performed in the world today.

There are other procedures, but those just mentioned are the basic ones.

Generally speaking, patients undergoing surgery are those who carry one hundred pounds or more of weight excess. Somewhat lower weights associated with significant comorbidities may qualify for WLS too.

The "one hundred pounds" number is the one medically accepted. That does not mean that insurance companies will always go along with it.

Corporate decisions are often capricious, arbitrary, unfair, discriminatory, and medically incorrect.

Figure 28. Normal Stomach

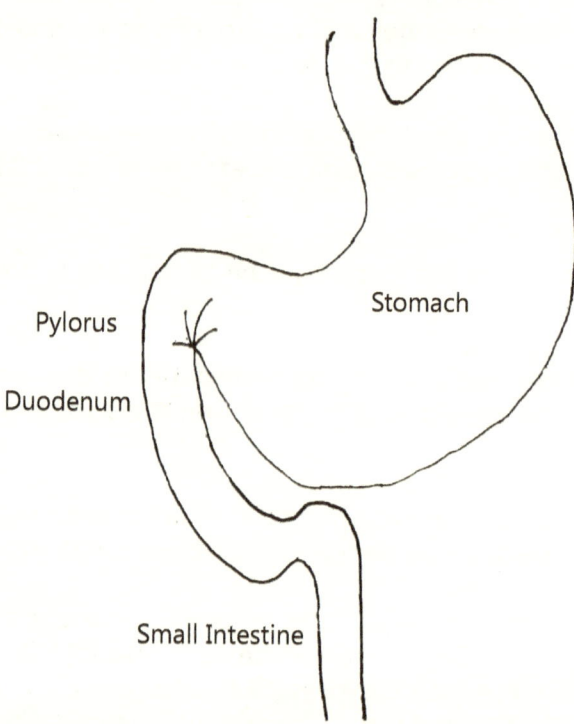

HOW DOES OBESITY SURGERY PRODUCE WEIGHT LOSS?

There are two general principles. Surgery works by

1. **restricting the amount of food that reaches the stomach** (*restrictive procedures*);
   This reduces the size of the stomach. The patient feels full quicker, so he/she eats less calories.
2. **restricting the amount of food that reaches the small bowel** (*malabsorptive procedures*).

1. RESTRICTIVE SURGERY

The size of the stomach is drastically reduced. A tiny stomach is made out of a large (normal) one.

There are three types of procedures:

- **Vertical banded gastroplasty (VBG)**
- **Adjustable gastric banding (AGB)**
- **Sleeve gastrectomy**

Vertical Banding Gastroplasty (VBG)

Surgeons consider this operation relatively easy to perform.

The stomach is stappled where the esophagus (food pipe) meets the stomach. The staples are placed vertically, and a plastic band is placed near the lower end of the staple line.

It is a purely restrictive procedure with no malabsorptive effect. It aims at restricting the patient's capacity to eat certain foods. The patient feels full after swallowing small amounts of food.

Advantages:
- It is reversible.
- No dumping occurs.
- The stomach anatomy is left intact.
- No nutritional deficiencies.

Disadvantages:
- The patient must be very disciplined and strict about diet limitations.
- Vomiting occurs if food is not adequately chewed or if food is eaten too quickly.

The operation produces a very small stomach (ten to thirty cubic centimeter in size = a shot glass). Note: a normal-size stomach holds four to six cups of food.

The constricting band restricts the amount of food that can leave the tiny pouch, and it keeps the outlet from stretching. There has been a decrease in the use of VBG since 1995.

Figure 29. Vertical-Banded Gastroplasty (VBG)

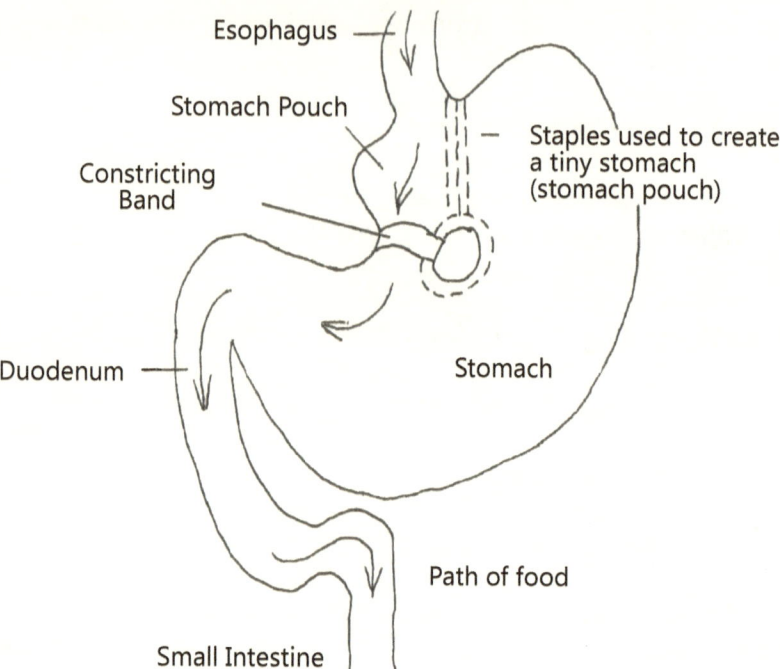

Adjustable Gastric Banding (AGB), also known as the Lap-Band

It is the least invasive of the purely restrictive bariatric surgical procedures.

It uses an inflatable silicone band to divide the stomach and create a small stomach pouch that can hold only a small amount of food. This band tightens the upper part of the stomach and leaves a pouch that contains ten to fifteen milliliter capacity. The lower, larger part of the stomach is below the band. These two parts are connected by a small outlet created by the band.

Food will get through the outlet—medically termed stoma—from the upper stomach pouch to the lower part, slowly, and the patient feels full for a longer period.

The band outlet's diameter can be adjusted to meet individual needs as the patient loses weight.

The inner layer of the band contains a balloon that can be inflated like a bicycle tire. It's left empty at the time of surgery. Thereafter, it's gradually filled with fluid (saline solution) by injection via a subcutaneous (under the skin) port or reservoir. This allows to modify the opening in the stomach after surgery. This maneuver can be done at the doctor's office.

The band is gradually tightened according to the patient's weight progress and satiety symptoms and provides progressive restriction that is adapted to each patient's needs.

The Lap-Band causes a slower and steadier weight loss than most other surgical procedures do. (Most obesity surgical procedures create very rapid weight loss.)

The Lap-Band system has been in use since the early mid-1990s, so there's no data on long-term outcomes.

Advantages:
- Simple operation and relatively safe.
- Faster recovery.
- Low incidence of major operative and postoperative complications.
- The stomach and the intestines are not open up or removed.
- The band is removable.
- The band is adjustable.

Disadvantages:
About 5 percent failure rate due to the following:
- Deep infection
- Band migration (slips out of position)
- Erosion into the stomach. (This does not create a serious problem but requires removal of the band.)
- Abnormal esophageal contractility that causes painful swallowing or reflux.
- Hardware malfunction: the band, the port, and the connection tubing are built to last for life. The port and the tube may break twist or become kinked. Reoperation may be required, but it's usually minor.
- Possible injuries to other organs during the operation—stomach, esophagus, liver, spleen—repair is done, and the operation is completed or abandoned, depending upon the surgeon's best judgment.

Figure 30. Adjustable Gastric Banding (AGB)

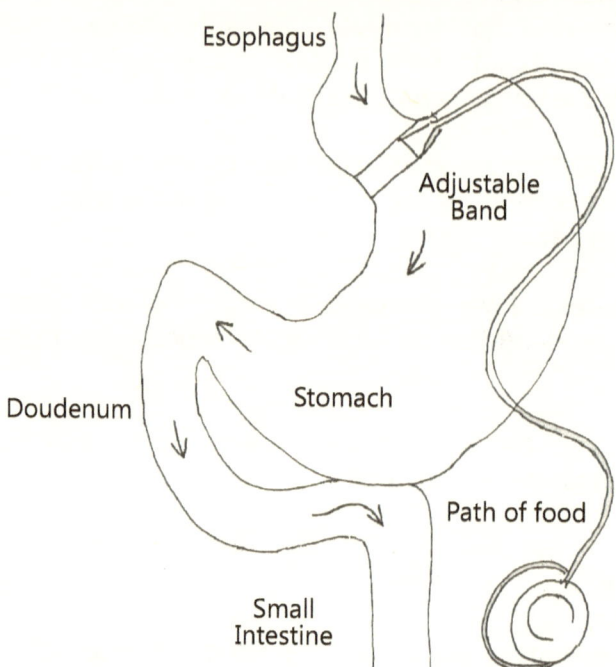

The two described procedures produce comparable results and a good initial weight loss. Since they work by restricting the amount of food in the stomach pouch and not by malabsorption, they have the advantage of not causing symptoms induced by the consumption of sugars, such as bloating, excessive abdominal gas, diarrhea.

Ironically, this "advantage" often turns to be an inconvenience. Since the patient is able to swallow sweets with impunity, he or she does, and sooner or later gains the weight back. In a ten-year period, about 80 percent of patients go back to their original weight, or very close to it.

C-SLEEVE (VERTICAL) GASTRECTOMY

This is an operation in which the stomach is divided lengthwise. A narrow, banana-shaped stomach tube (sleeve) is created by removing 80 percent or more of the stomach. This results in a smaller stomach, which restricts the amount of food that can be eaten at any given time.

A camera and small instruments are placed through small holes in the abdomen. The instruments cuts and staples the stomach, and the unused portion is removed.

The procedure takes about thirty minutes and has been reported to produce a 50 percent or higher excess weight loss. Results as far as improvement of diabetes, hypertension, sleep apnea after sleeve gastrectomy are comparable to those of other restrictive operations.

The sleeve gastrectomy is usually performed as the first stage of biliopancreatic diversion with duodenal switch in patients who may be at high risk from more extensive types of surgery. This method does not affect the absorption of food. It simply reduces significantly the size of the stomach. Most of it is removed. That leads to decreased production of a hormone called ghrelin. This, in turn, may reduce hunger more than other purely restrictive operations such as the gastric band.

Figure 31. Sleeve Gastrectomy

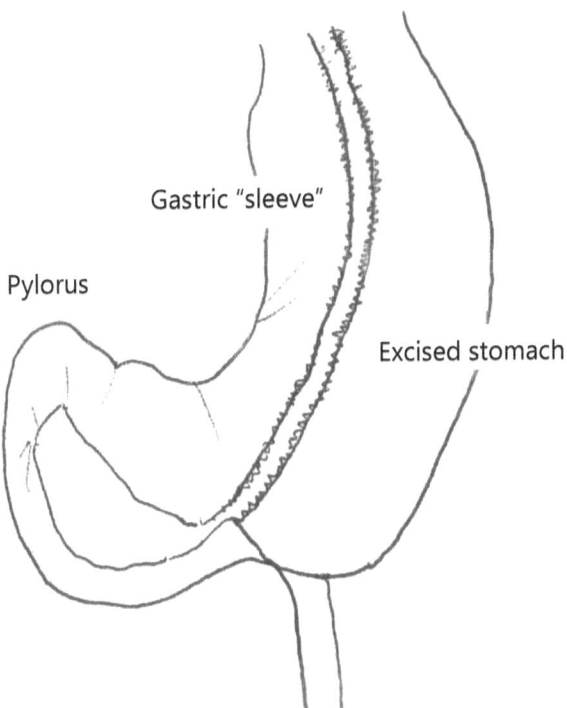

Gastric "sleeve"

Pylorus

Excised stomach

2. MALABSORPTIVE SURGERY

Biliopancreatic Diversion with Duodenal Switch Procedure (BPD/DS)

This is a more complicated malabsorptive operation. Portions of the stomach are removed.

The small pouch that remains is connected directly to the final segment of the small intestine, completely bypassing most of the intestine.

The size of the stomach is reduced but modestly so. Because this bypass isolates most of the gut, the digestive enzymes and bile only mix with the swallowed food in a tiny portion at the end of the intestine, producing an ineffective absorption and significant weight loss.

This procedure helps most people to achieve 75-80 percent loss of their excessive weight and maintain that loss long-term.

Unfortunately, substantial side effects and complications limit the usefulness and application of this method. It is much less frequently used than the gastric bypass operation, but it finds its application in selective cases.

Advantages:
* Better eating quality when compared to other WLS operations. Patient may eat "more normally" and still achieve excellent long-term weight loss,—75 percent to 80 percent loss of their excessive weight and maintain that loss long-term.
* Essentially avoids the dumping syndrome.

Disadvantages:
* Greater probability of chronic diarrhea.
* Significant malabsorption component. Nutrients, vitamins, minerals, and protein deficiencies are common. The latter is the most serious potential complication of malabsorption and may be serious enough to require hospitalization for intravenous replenishment.
* Need to take supplemental calcium and vitamins, particularly vitamin D, lifelong.

Patients need *very close* and careful lifelong *medical supervision and follow-up.*

Pregnancy should be avoided. This operation should ideally be performed in women who have completed their childbearing.

*Rapid passage of food from the stomach into the gut causes diarrhea, foul-smelling stools, and increased flatus. (This results from incomplete indigestion.)

Because of the listed disadvantages, the BPD/DS is not frequently used, and many bariatric surgeons have abandoned this procedure altogether.

3. COMBINATION OF RESTRICTIVE AND MALABSORPTIVE SURGERY

Roux-en-Y (RYGBP)

This is currently the preferred and most commonly used bariatric surgical intervention in the United States and worldwide. It is a combination of restrictive and malabsorptive methods.

It is restrictive because the size of the stomach is reduced.

Some surgeons, though, create a small pouch that is shaped to be about the size of your thumb and will hold 20 milliliters or less. In these cases, the stomach pouch is even smaller than a shot glass and will restrict food to two to three tiny bites. This restriction is one of the ways gastric bypass leads to weight loss.

A portion of the stomach is sectioned off, creating a small pouch that allows reduced food intake (restrictive component).

The malabsorptive component comes from bypassing a small portion of the beginning of the intestine together with most of the stomach.

The intestine usually cannot easily handle high concentrations of sugars. When a meal with heavy sugar content is ingested, the patient may experience nausea, vomiting, diarrhea, bloating, and dizziness, the so-called dumping syndrome.

The dumping syndrome is certainly very uncomfortable. Trying to avoid it, the patient restricts sugar consumption. This, in turn, means reduced caloric intake.

Food then will avoid passage through the duodenum and part of the jejunum, thereby limiting its absorption. Digestive juices and bile will drain in the duodenum as usual, but these will not meet the ingested food until they become in touch with each other in a more advanced section of the jejunum farther down.

Advantages:
* Good results
* Considered to be generally safe
* Low incidence of complications
* Very good control of food intake
* Dumping syndrome stimulates patient to avoid sweets consumption.
* The procedure is to be considered permanent. However, it can be reversed if needed.

Disadvantages:
* Failure of the staple line
* Ulcers
* Narrowing/blockage of the stoma
* Vomiting if food is eaten too quickly or not chewed properly

This procedure is effective, carries a low incidence of complications, and it is also considered safe.

High Glycemic Index and What It Means

Foods that are rapidly converted into sugar (glucose) are said to have a high glycemic index (ice creams, cookies, chocolate, potatoes, white rice, white bread, high sugar cereals) and are prone to cause nausea, vomiting, and diarrhea.

Dumping is more severe during the first year after surgery. Then improves, but it never completely disappears.

Figure 32. Roux-en-Y

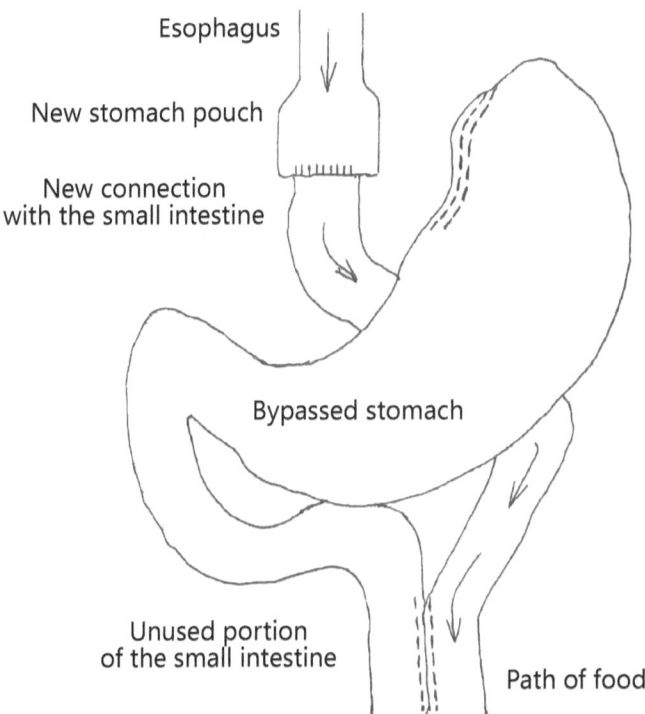

Esophagus

New stomach pouch

New connection
with the small intestine

Bypassed stomach

Unused portion
of the small intestine

Path of food

TECHNICAL APPROACH TO BARIATRIC SURGERY

These operations can be accomplished by different approaches:

1. Traditional long midabdominal incision

2. Minimally invasive surgery (laparoscopic surgery)

Minimally, invasive surgery (laparoscopic surgery) minimizes the incision's length, reduces trauma, pain, and postoperative recovery time. Typically, patients leave the hospital on the second postoperative day.

There are a number of operations designed to achieve weight loss. We are not mentioning them here because they have not been proven to be very effective or are associated with frequent undesirable side effects.

In both normal and gastric bypass patients, nutrients are absorbed in the small intestine.

In the most widely performed gastric bypass operation (Roux-en-Y), bile and pancreatic juice mix with nutrients, and these get absorbed. The acid production by the lower part of the stomach helps the digestion of bulky meals.

The bypassed stomach and small intestine play vital roles in the absorption of iron, calcium, and vitamin B12. Patients must always take these substances, and their blood levels must be periodically checked.

How does the bypassed lower part of the stomach react?

Since the blood supply is not altered during the gastric resection, the stomach remains healthy. This lower stomach portion manufactures a substance called intrinsic factor, which is essential for the absorption of vitamin B12 by the small intestine.

Staples and MRI

The staples placed on the stomach and the intestines are of much smaller size than the staples used to close a skin wound.

Each staple is a tiny piece of stainless steel or titanium. These components render the staples totally inert in the body. MRI testing will not affect them.

You can also get through an airport metal detector without activating the alarm.

Comparison between the Roux-en-Y Gastric Bypass and Lap-Band

Roux-en-Y Gastric Bypass	Lap-Band
Preferred, most frequently used method	Selectively acceptable new technology
Weight loss is rapid.	Weight loss is slow and steady.
Usually, 70 percent of excess weight is lost in	Usually, about 60

the first year after surgery	percent of excess weight is lost in three years after surgery.
Mineral deficiency is due to malabsorption.	Mineral deficiency is due to reduced food consumption.

Long-term multivitamins and minerals supplementation is recommended for both.

Dumping syndrome (intolerance to sugar and some carbohydrates), which helps patients to stay away from sugars.	No dumping syndrome.
May be reversed.	May be reversed.
No plastic material is used.	Plastic material is used.
	The band needs to be adjusted for best results, usually every month the first year after surgery.

When a patient is *not* a good candidate for Lap-Band surgery:

* Severe GERD or gastroesophageal reflux or esophageal motor abnormalities
* Prior stomach surgery
* Home is located more than four hours' drive from the surgeon. The band needs close follow-up and access to the surgeon.

IMPLANTABLE GASTRIC STIMULATION SYSTEM (IGS)

A battery pack is implanted under the skin, and a wire connects the battery to the stomach. Electrical discharges stimulate the stomach vagus nerve. This results in decreased gastrointestinal contractions.

The surgeon tests the patient by delivering currents that produce nausea. Then he/she decreases the voltage until the patient states that he/she is not hungry.

Different degrees of electrical stimulation are applied to determine which proves to be the most effective in reducing appetite.

This is a new procedure and is still under investigation. Its advantage is its simplicity and lack of complications or mortality. It does not appear though to induce a major weight loss, but it may be considered when other procedures have failed. The intended weight loss is less than one hundred pounds, or it is desirable to stimulate some weight loss in preparation for one of the standard weight-loss operations.

A NEW IDEA: OBESITY SURGERY THAT REQUIRES NO TRADITIONAL SURGERY

Brigham and Women's Hospital is offering the possibility of a safer, less traumatic operation to deal with morbid obesity. Dr. Christopher Thompson, director of bariatric endoscopy at Brigham, is the principal researcher in a clinical trial that is underway. The procedure consists in introducing a tube through the patient's mouth and down the throat and then use a tiny needle to sew a series of pleats in the stomach. The pleats narrow the stomach, and this is unable to accept regular amounts of food.

This procedure replaces the bariatric methods that cut the patient's abdomen. Since it is less invasive, the researchers hope that infections, bleeding, and scarring could be avoided.

It is estimated that several years will be needed to learn whether this innovative procedure is safe or effective enough to be offered to the public.

WEIGHT LOSS FOLLOWING BARIATRIC SURGERY

Weight loss with the Roux-en-Y procedure usually reaches 65 percent to 75 percent of a person's excess weight within the first year. By this time, the stomach had time to stretch a bit and allows more food. Exercise, diet, discipline, restrain, and method will help to keep the weight off.

Most—but not all patients—who had the Roux-en-Y operation maintain a good weight for a period of five years.

There's rapid weight loss in the first six months after the operation. The stomach is swollen from the surgical trauma, and the appetite is gone. Initially, you'll only drink liquids, but when you start eating real food, the weight loss will slow down. The appetite returns in about six months.

IMPORTANCE OF CHARACTER, MOTIVATION, AND CONSISTENCY

If a person is unable to radically change his or her lifestyle, follow up a lifelong program of adequate and selective nutritional guidelines, regular exercises, greatly improves or suppresses compulsions, character flaws, personality disorder, or psychological dysfunctions, surgical treatment of morbid obesity is not recommended.

The surgeon looks for the ideal patient as much as the patient looks for the ideal surgeon.

Some patients will say, "I have some coworkers and a couple of relatives who had gastric bypass, and they are not doing well. In fact, they're very unhappy! They've gained their weight back. That's the reason why I don't want to go through this kind of treatment!"

Carefully questioned, this person admitted that those who gained their weight back did not follow postoperative instructions the way they should have.

The best bariatric surgeon in the world will not be able to help you unless you help yourself.

Bariatric surgery extends you a hand. It gives you a chance to become a different and healthier person. But it will only work if you do your part, and only if you do it consistently and permanently.

THE MOMENT OF TRUTH

Unquestionably, the decision to undergo WLS is a major one, and one of the most transcendent decisions you'll make in the course of your life.

Talking to people who already had WLS will give you a better sense about expectations.

One suggestion: When you are told "my sister died from this kind of surgery," do more research and find out, if at all possible who performed the operation and where it was done. Stories like these usually originated at a time when bariatric surgical methods were less perfected and/or the surgeon who performed the operation wasn't an expert on the field.

In obesity surgery, as much as in any other medical area, successful treatments are directly proportional to the *quality* of the medical care.

Surgery may indeed cause serious complications, death included, and these may happen with the best surgeon and at the best hospital. All you can hope for, and expect, if you have selected an excellent professional, is a low incidence and a low probability of complications.

Left untouched to its own slow motion, stubborn pace, morbid obesity carries a greater risk than the operations designed to correct it.

No one in this world can assure you success with *any* form of treatment. All doctors can do for you is explain the pros and cons of various treatment alternatives.

Risks are always present, no matter what you do. *So when you approach the treatment options of morbid obesity—surgery versus no surgery—you've got to consider where your risks are higher.*

Then it is up to you, and no one else, to decide what course to take.

That's the way it is. And that's the way it should be.

CHAPTER 7

RISKS, INCONVENIENCIES, AND BENEFITS OF BARIATRIC SURGERY

In the practice of medicine, there are good treatments and bad treatments, never perfect treatments.

The risks of serious medical events are a great concern in morbidly obese patients who are not treated with bariatric surgery and those who undergo the operation. The big issue is, which are the lesser ones and what's the best time to take them.

This is not the right place to review the history of mankind's great medical achievements, but I'd like to say this much: every progress made in the art and science of healing since the beginning of times has carried with it an abundance of pain, some inspiration, plenty of perspiration and hard work, extraordinary vicissitudes, and an inordinate amount of human suffering.

Countless medical and surgical treatments resulted in failure before they became successful. Same thing happened with nonmedical inventions: take the case of the famous Swedish inventor Alfred Nobel.

Nobel was a chemist and patented nitroglycerine in 1867 under the name Dynamite. No sooner had the young scientist begun mass production of nitroglycerin than an explosion ripped through the plant, killing five people.

Explosions apart, dynamite became a huge success, and Nobel amassed a fortune today worth approximately 520 million dollars, which after his death in 1896 was used to endow the annual Nobel Prize.

I only mention this here to make a point: human progress never takes an easy road. And in the practice of medicine, treatments, procedures, and operations that finally made it to the top and reached the pinnacle of their prestige never offered 100 percent guarantee of success.

It is indeed *possible* to have an operation without complications, but the *possibility* of complications always exists.

Still, in highly competent hands, the surgical treatment of morbid obesity is generally safe, and in properly selected patients, the operation is usually well tolerated, and the risks of surgery are less than the risks of continuing with morbid obesity.

WHY SOME DOCTORS ADVISE PATIENTS AGAINST WLS

a. Bias, prejudice, and negative feelings toward the obese. Prejudicial behavior and attitudes are common in our culture. Physicians are part of that culture.
b. Lack of familiarity with the subject.
c. Insufficient exposure to cases of morbid obesity. Very few such clients are part of the practitioner's practice.
d. The physician has outdated information about the new, safer, and more effective methods and techniques deployed in obesity surgery.
e. Unawareness about the selection of Centers of Excellence (COE) by the Surgical Review Corporation (SRC).

    The identification of COE across the United States allows patients to consult surgeons who have been recognized by the Surgical Review Corporation (SRC) for their superior skills and not just good but excellent results.

f. Fear of losing a contractual arrangement with a HMO because the recommended WLS is not considered a cost-effective decision.

NEGATIVE ASPECTS OF WEIGHT-LOSS SURGERY (WLS)

1. WLS will not produce good results unless you radically change your lifestyle and make a permanent commitment to adhere to an appropriate diet, regular exercise, and the recommended follow-up.
2. You'll have to be very careful about taking the necessary vitamins and supplements to avoid nutritional deficiencies.
3. It is not true that you'll never feel deprived. Sometimes, you will.

4. To lose a lot of weight will create a gastrointestinal imbalance and unpleasant symptoms, which would have never existed without surgery.
5. Some complications from surgery, such as the need for immediate reoperation (due to leakage of gastric juice and germs into the abdominal cavity) or delayed reoperation (due to intestinal obstruction) may occur.
6. Rapid substantial weight loss following surgery may cause serious, and even life-threatening cardiac arrhythmias.
7. You'll never be able to eat junk foods again (cookies, pastries, ice cream, cakes, chips, and others).
8. Weight gain following gastroplasty usually results from gradual stretching and enlargement of the gastric pouch or the narrow outlet, both resulting from the consumption of the wrong foods.
9. If you question your determination to make the right decisions following bariatric surgery, you're not ready for this kind of treatment.
10. Substantial weight loss following WLS at times leads to redundant, prominent, hanging skin folds in different parts of the body that can only be corrected by plastic surgery.

Now the fact that you are not ready for WLS at one particular time does not mean that you will not be able to radically change that position in the future.

A TYPICAL EXAMPLE OF A PATIENT WHO DOES NOT QUALIFY FOR WLS

A forty-year-old female, with a weight of 340 pounds and a height of five feet five, told me that under no circumstances she would be willing to "sacrifice" her eating habits, no matter how great the risk of sudden death, heart attacks, cancer, and other illnesses.

She said, *"I like food. Actually, I'm not totally sincere when I say that! The truth is that I love food! I really do. I enjoy eating all kinds of foods at any time and every time I want. And that makes me a very happy person. You're telling me that I have to restrict myself for the rest of my life? Doctor, you don't know who you're talking to. I'd never do that. I don't care if I die tomorrow. But in the meantime, I'm having a ball. I don't mean to be rude to you. You've been kind to me. So please don't be offended by what I'm gonna tell you now: this whole idea of changing my gut and end eating like a little bird . . . sucks! It really does. I want no part of that!"*

Well . . . that's it! That way of thinking excluded her from any consideration of obesity surgery.

A TYPICAL EXAMPLE OF SOMEONE WHO HAD WLS AND SHOULD HAVE NEVER HAD IT

A seventy-two-year-old lady carried 220 pounds of weight excess. Years ago, she had gastric banding first. No results. Years later, she had gastric bypass surgery: no results. She said to me, "These operations are not good. I've followed the doctor's instructions, ate the right food, but I never lost any significant amount of weight and remained morbidly obese for the rest of my life."

Her husband (also a very obese individual) interrupted her and stated that she was the only one responsible for the treatment failure and described how poorly she had followed the nutritionist and physicians' instructions. And said, "We, and I mean both of us, always ate the wrong food, and we still do! I'm sorry to say, my wife is not telling the truth!"

She finally admitted her husband was correct. Evidently, denial was part of her problem.

Denial is a defense mechanism that protects against anxiety. We don't like a problem, so we pretend it doesn't exist.

SOME RISKS OF WEIGHT-LOSS SURGERY

- Allergic reactions to medications
- Spleen or other organs injuries
- Difficulties into recognizing abdominal catastrophe
- Anesthesia complications
- Bleeding
- Pneumonia
- Respiratory failure
- Infections (bladder, skin, wound, lung, deep abdominal)
- Leaking of stomach acid, bacteria, and digestive enzymes into the abdominal cavity
- Ulcers and narrowing of the connection between the stomach and the small bowel
- Bowel obstruction
- Lactose intolerance

- Malabsorption of nutrients, minerals, and vitamins (this can be prevented if patient follows medical recommendations)
- Medications side effects
- Cardiac events
- Abdominal wall hernia
- Hair loss (a frequent short-term problem)
- Pregnancy and possible fetal complications may occur for one year following the operation
- Leg blood clots (DVT or deep venous thrombosis)
- Pulmonary emboli (clots from the legs or thighs traveling to the lungs)
- Sudden death
- Depression and psychological stress
- Marital and relationship problems
- Death

Dumping Syndrome

After gastric bypass, one of the key elements that help a patient control calorie intake is the fact that the constructed tiny stomach pouch drains food into a portion of the small bowel called the jejunum.

The jejunum is naturally not made to handle concentrated calories, particularly refined sugar. So if you consume sugar following this surgery—such as soda, chocolate, candy, ice cream—a reaction will take place. That is called dumping. You will experience tachycardia (fast heart rate), will be clammy and will perspire profusely, and will have acute abdominal cramps, diarrhea, and weakness for a while.

Dumping is not a dangerous event, but it makes a person feel so miserable, that in a way, helps him/her to avoid sugar consumption.

Patients who undergo treatment with the adjustable gastric band do not have dumping.

Lactose Intolerance

Lactose is a type of sugar found in milk and dairy products. Absorption of lactose requires a particular enzyme that mostly exists in the bypassed portion of intestine. So some patients who never had lactose intolerance before surgery will experience abdominal cramps and flatulence (excessive amount of abdominal gas) after gastric bypass. An over-the-counter medication, Lactaid, is helpful.

Usually, and due to bowel adaptation, lactose intolerance symptoms improved six months following the operation.

Mineral Absorption

The bypassed segments of the GI (gastrointestinal) tract, namely, the lower part of the stomach and the upper part of the small intestine, due to the created surgical exclusion, do not participate in the digestion of food.

These segments of the GI tube play an important role in the absorption of iron, calcium, magnesium, vitamin B12, and to a lesser degree B6.

Patients who had gastric bypass surgery should be on lifelong regimen of multivitamins, iron, and calcium (usually calcium citrate).

Although patients treated with an adjustable gastric band do not have deficient absorption of the mentioned vitamins and minerals, they badly need these nutrients because of their overall poor intake of these substances.

DVT (Deep Venous Thrombosis) and PE (Pulmonary Emboli)

Sometimes, deep veins' clot formation takes place during the operation. Prevention is attempted with leg compression stockings and subcutaneous heparin (blood thinner). These measures are implemented until the patient is discharged from the hospital. Another very important preventive measure is getting the patient mobilized and out of bed as soon as possible after the operation.

The Stomach Pouch Inflammation

The stomach pouch has a capacity of one ounce or less. During the first months after surgery, it is rather stiff due to surgically induced inflammation. From six to twelve months following the operation, the pouch expands a little bit and becomes more pliable. In the end, the capacity of the pouch grows to have a meal capacity larger than at the beginning.

The Question of Being Hungry Following Gastric Bypass

In general, patients have poor appetite for the first four to six weeks after surgery. Appetite, then, gradually returns, but it is not excessive.

Make sure you don't mix fluids with solid food since the liquid washes food out of the pouch. If the food passes too fast through the pouch, then your appetite will be greater, and that is exactly what you do not want to happen. Wait thirty minutes between solid and liquid foods.

Excess Skin

Morbid obesity stretches the skin. Unfortunately, once the skin is stretched, sometimes, it refuses to shrink. Some patients are left with prominent floppy areas of skin, more so in the abdomen, upper arms, thighs, and breasts.

The size of the skin folds varies considerably from person to person. Exercise will not correct this problem. Plastic surgery will.

Skin surgery for removal of excess skin should be delayed up until the time you reached the desired weight. Doing otherwise means to develop additional folds after corrective skin surgery. More flabby skin will continue to appear as long as you continue to lose weight. That's not good. Wait until you're done with your weight excess, and you've stabilized it.

Hair Loss

Three to five months following gastric bypass surgery, most patients notice an increase in hair loss. This is the result of abrupt calorie and protein deficit that occurs after surgery.

Hair loss can be modest or alarming. Some patients lose big chunks of hair and become annoyed and preoccupied about this. That improves one year after surgery and one and one-half year following the operation, the hair is back.

To increase protein intake, you should eat more frequently (three meals a day) and only healthy food.

Gallstones

Patients who have cycles of weight loss and weight gain are predisposed to gallstones formation. Morbid obesity has a high incidence of gallstone formation and so does rapid weight loss. Mechanisms responsible for gallstone formation include increased biliary secretion of cholesterol and increased retention of bile within the gallbladder that follow bariatric surgery. A daily dose of five hundred milligrams of ursodeoxycholic acid in divided doses semidaily for six months is effective prophylaxis for gallstone formation.

Depression and Psychological Stress

Some morbidly obese patients suffer from addiction to food. There are people who control the food addiction but trade one addiction for another and get involved with alcohol, drugs, or gambling.

Psychotherapy helps. So do the medications for anxiety depression or bipolar disorders. Some mental disorders (bipolar disease is just an example) are sometimes important contributors to morbid obesity.

Following successful gastric bypass surgery and appropriate psychiatric management, a couple of years later, when the patient lost two hundred pounds of excess weight, he/she may be prescribed another psychotropic drug that induces a voracious appetite as a side effect. This situation requires quick intervention to replace it with another drug that does not significantly alter the patient's appetite.

Marital and Relationship Problems

Gastric bypass and the dramatic weight loss that follows it affect a relationship. It is preferable to start thinking about these changes in advance, even before surgery. This may or may not help the quality of the relationship, but at least, you're not going to be taken by surprise or overreact to situations that unfold as the weight loss progresses.

Experts in relationships remind us that most relationships don't work. Or they don't work very well. Or they don't work for too long. And I'm not referring to cases of morbid obesity but the general population. The often higher than 50 percent divorce rate we see in the United States provides the evidence.

The percentage of couples who divorce in the two years that follow WLS is high. In some cases, marital or relationship counseling helps.

Factors that increase the risks of WLS:

- Super morbid obesity, BMI > 50
- Concomitant heart disease or other important disease or organ failure (e.g., kidney, liver, blood disorders, lungs)
- Severe ambulatory difficulties (use of walker or scooter)
- History of smoking
- Chronic obstructive lung disease
- Recent or current therapy with steroids
- Past blood clot in legs (deep venous thrombosis or DVT) or pulmonary emboli

BENEFITS OF SUCCESSFUL WEIGHT-LOSS SURGERY

The successful treatment of morbid obesity is followed by very substantial improvement or resolution of its numerous comorbidities, including most cases of pseudotumor cerebri, metabolic syndrome, polycystic ovarian syndrome, hirsutism, menstrual irregularities, asthma, respiratory function, obstructive sleep apnea, type 2 diabetes, venous stasis disease of the lower extremities, skin infections, hypertension, dyslipidemia, reversion of infertility, reflux esophagitis, nonalcoholic fatty liver disease, better outlook for postoperative complications following any kind of major surgery, cardiovascular disease, including the incidence of strokes, myocardial infarctions, congestive heart failure, premature death, and sudden death.

Also resolved or greatly improved are cases of stress urinary incontinence, gout, migraine, depression, and degenerative joint disease symptoms affecting hips, knees, ankles, and lower spine.

An individual who has normalized his/her weight feels like a new person. And that means a new life. There's a self-esteem boost, the feeling of being in control, finds him/herself more assertive, has more mental and physical energy, renewed social, employment, and personal relationships opportunities. He/she is no longer the object of discrimination, prejudice, or demeaning attitudes. Practices regular exercises and sports and is able to take on challenging and gratifying social and professional activities.

The quality of life improves in 95 percent of patients. According to a recent study from the Agency for Healthcare Research and Quality (AHRQ), the mortality rate associated with bariatric surgery dropped from 0.89 percent in 1998 to 0.19 percent in 2004, and the mortality rate from obesity was reduced by 89 percent after bariatric surgery according to a study published in the *Annals of Surgery* in 2004.

Now let's see the other side of the coin, and the problems that surface when the morbidly obese patient requires WLS and doesn't get it.

CHAPTER 8

RISKS FROM UNTREATED MORBID OBESITY

Anything we do—or we don't do—carries a risk.

Some of the weight-loss surgical complications may cause disability and loss of life as we mentioned in the preceding chapter. Notably, some of the same dangerous listed complications, such as myocardial infarction, heart failure, stroke, respiratory failure, and sudden death occur more often in morbidly obese patients who remain untreated.

Morbid obesity is defined as one hundred pounds above ideal body weight, or a BMI of forty or more. As the BMI increases, so does the mortality rate from all causes, especially from cardiovascular disease.

Cardiovascular disease incidence is 50 percent to 100 percent higher than that of individuals who have a BMI of twenty-five.

There are potential complications of obesity surgery, but when the operation is performed by a very competent and experienced surgeon, their incidence is low.

On the other hand, consider the risks of other common complications of untreated obesity, such as an acute myocardial infarction. This is a serious illness that carries 30 percent mortality. (The first acute myocardial infarction in women may be fatal in 40-50 percent of cases). Forty to seventy-five percent of all victims die before reaching the hospital. Forty-two percent of women die within a year of an acute heart attack in the United States. Twenty-four percent of men die within a year of a heart attack (the National Women's Health Information Center, CDC).

Strokes, congestive heart failure, life-threatening cardiac rhythm disturbances, and acute pulmonary embolus—all of them frequent disorders experienced by morbidly obese patients are responsible for many premature demises.

Hypertension and diabetes are two serious ailments characteristically suffered by patients with morbid obesity. Any of these two disorders is responsible for higher incidence of strokes, myocardial infarctions, poor cardiac muscle functioning (congestive heart failure), and advanced renal failure that may require dialysis and/or kidney transplantation. Diabetes alone may lead to blindness, leg amputations, carotid artery blockage, arterial disease of the lower extremities, neuropathy, and sexual dysfunction.

Morbidly obese patients frequently suffer from migraines, airway disease, nonalcoholic fatty liver disease, the metabolic syndrome, high cholesterol and triglycerides blood levels, venous disease of the lower extremities, lymphedema, reflux esophagitis (acid going from the stomach to the esophagus causing heartburn), Barrett's esophagus, a condition characterized by abnormal cells in the esophagus that predisposes to esophageal cancer, gallstones, higher incidence of various other cancers.

Urinary incontinence (or bowel incontinence) is common and results from increased intra-abdominal pressure (overflow urinary incontinence). Anal incontinence may also occur although it seems to be less frequent.

Degenerative joint disease of the lumbar spine and knees, at times of disabling proportions, polycystic ovarian syndrome with menstrual irregularities and hirsutism (excessive hair growth outside the normal areas of the body) and depression.

Occasionally, a condition called pseudotumor cerebri presents with severe headaches and, at times, blindness. The cause of this disease is not known, but it's upsetting enough to ruin a person's life.

And there are many more illnesses that can be added to this gloomy list: infertility, dangerous effects on pregnancy for the mother and the fetus, increased tendency to infections and disorders of the blood coagulation, delayed recovery following accidents, sexual dysfunctions, psychosocial complications, skin diseases, periodontitis (inflammation and infection of the gums).

The possibility of sudden death in the morbidly obese is an ever-present risk, even in the absence of an identifiable cardiac dysfunction.

The Framingham study specifically demonstrated a sixfold to twelvefold excess mortality rate in morbidly obese men.

Obesity is associated with a low-grade diffuse inflammatory state evidenced by elevated blood levels of proinflammatory substances, such as C-reactive protein, cytokines, interleukin-6, which contribute to the damage of the arteries and their eventual blockage.

Respiratory insufficiency is due to deficient lung expansion (called hypoventilation). Obstructive sleep apnea due to obstruction of the upper respiratory airway, with its disturbed sleep and snoring at night and somnolence during the day.

There are ailments that doctors easily diagnose in the slim patient but find it more difficult to diagnose in the severely obese: peritonitis, pancreatitis, diverticulitis, and abdominal infections may be catastrophic in the obese. One of the reasons for unfavorable outcomes of acute abdominal crises in the morbidly obese is that acute intra-abdominal illnesses are more difficult to diagnose than in normal-weight patients.

The morbidly obese is at a higher risk of dying than other patients with treatable infections.

Many authorities feel that WLS is particularly warranted and more urgently needed when morbid obesity is associated with type 2 diabetes, severe degenerative joint disease causing serious limitations and disability, moderate to severe sleep apnea, pseudotumor cerebri, polycystic ovarian syndrome not responsive to a medication called metformin, severe gastroesophageal reflux or Barrett's esophagus, and nonalcoholic steatohepatitis.

The success rate in treating morbid obesity by drugs, diet, exercise, hypnosis, jaw wiring, voluntary incarceration, intragastric balloons have been proven to have a very high rate of failure.

About 95 percent of patients who have been treated by weight-reduction programs regain all the weight they lost within two years of the onset of therapy.

To sum it up:

Risks exist whatever course you choose to follow, and that is, weight-loss surgery versus no surgery; but *the incidence of obesity surgery serious complications in excellent hands is* low, *and the incidence of serious and fatal complications of untreated morbid obesity is* high.

Careful medical and surgical evaluation and consultations, when necessary, with a lung specialist, cardiologist, or other needed professionals *will determine how high or low risks are for you, either by avoiding WLS or by having it.*

Once the facts and probabilities are clearly explained to you by your team of specialists, it will be up to you to decide.

It's never an easy decision. Nevertheless, it's one that, at one point and, hopefully, sooner than later, you'll have to face.

CHAPTER 9

REACTIONS OF FRIENDS AND RELATIVES TO YOUR SUCCESS (BE PREPARED, JUST IN CASE)

There's always a price we pay for failure and success.

I'm not a psychologist, and I don't want to convey you the impression that I'm trying to act like one.

I do want, though, to offer you personal observations on human behavior in relation to the morbid obesity issue, and the repercussions that occasionally follow successful weight-loss surgery.

I'd also like to submit to you that you do not have to be a certified psychotherapist to know that there are wonderful, caring, generous, and sensitive people and also individuals who are mean, jealous, vicious, insecure, and disturbingly stupid.

If you ever become successful in normalizing your weight, you are going to look very different than you did in the past. I've seen a number of men and women who looked absolutely beautiful after normalizing their weight.

That is a wonderful achievement, and one that you should be proud of. It takes considerable courage and hard work to get there.

This success of yours is capable of making some people nervous. These individuals may be just acquaintances or coworkers, but some could be your closest friends or relatives, individuals whom you've known, trusted, and even loved very dearly for decades, if not a lifetime.

The dramatic improvement of your physical appearance associated with an increased assertiveness and self-confidence may evoke reactions of jealousy, envy, and other previously disguised or hidden psychological dysfunctions or personality disorders. These may translate into ungracious thoughts, feelings, and behavior.

I recently saw a woman who had gastric bypass surgery a couple of years prior and looked stunning. Her successful obesity surgery changed her personality. She found herself very secure and confident. Her husband used to put her down with abusive verbal barrages. When he saw that he couldn't dominate and control her any longer (the psychologist explained to me), he sued for divorce.

When she suffered from morbid obesity, she felt diminished and unable to confront her husband. But with the normalization of her weight and her new and very attractive physical appearance, she was ready to challenge her husband's abuse and gladly gave him the divorce. *She told me, "I regret nothing. I have a wonderful new life now!"*

Imagine this other scenario: you've lost one hundred or two hundred pounds or whatever, and you're going to be elated about it.

If one of your friends or relatives suffers from morbid obesity and has been unable to match that kind of performance, he or she may resent it. Frustration prevails.

Initially, his or her attitude may be pleasant and polite, but you may soon notice that on your birthday, you'll get no greeting card although you had been getting them from that person for the past fifteen years.

Another time, you may be told something like this: "True, you did well, but you could have done better!"

Or simply, he or she may contact you to say hello once in a blue moon when, previously, that happened three times a week.

Some dysfunctional characters can't enjoy or even witness other people's happiness. They are unable to get rid of or deal with their anger and negative emotions. Your success reminds them of their failure. Your achievement opens wounds that drain their character flaws and insecurities. You represent the fulfillment and joy that they couldn't reach.

You are going to be physically, psychologically, and emotionally in better shape than they will. Socially and professionally, you'll advance your agenda and experience some gains too.

These tormented souls can be pretty toxic, particularly if you allow them to use you as a punching bag.

It's human nature. Many such characters pollute the world and exist at all socioeconomic, cultural, and educational levels.

You should be prepared for such reactions. Don't be shocked if you see some of your "dear friends" ventilating their frustration in an open or a camouflaged, passive-aggressive, convoluted way.

And now, the good news. Your achievement will evoke true happiness and joy in those who *truly* love you. They will rejoice seeing you the way you are and will sincerely share your happiness.

Just watch out for those who may not be so receptive or sympathetic to your triumph and come to accept the fact that some "friendships" were not meant to be.

Of course, there are wonderful people in this world. You'll just have to work a little harder to find them.

CHAPTER 10

A CONVERSATION WITH TWO PROMINENT BARIATRIC SURGEONS

For a number of years, I had the privilege of sharing patients' consultations and care with two masters of the field of obesity surgery. That's the way I learned how successful the surgical approach of morbid obesity can be.

In this chapter, they answer my questions about issues related to obesity surgery. I think it's interesting and also intriguing to learn what's going on in the minds of two surgeons who excel in the practice of their profession.

Robert T. Marema, M.D., F.A.C.S., is C.E.O., U.S. Bariatric, medical director of bariatrics, Holy Cross Hospital, Fort Lauderdale, Florida, and medical director of bariatrics, Florida Hospital, Celebration Health, Orlando, Florida.

Carlos Carrasquilla, M.D., F.A.C.S., is director of Surgical Weight Loss Institute, University Hospital, Tamarac, Florida, and director of Surgical Institute for Weight Control, Fort Lauderdale, Florida.

CHAPUNOFF: I've been looking forward to this conversation for some time. Sharing your thoughts and experience is a great privilege for me, and I appreciate your gesture more than I can say.

Some of the issues I'm going to raise are sensitive and provocative, and they will make some people uncomfortable. Nevertheless, if discussing them will result in increased awareness of the problems faced by the morbidly obese, and we can transmit that information to those affected—health care practitioners and the general population—and if, in some way, we contribute to change the attitude of some health insurance corporations that display disdain and indifference for the well-being and survival of severely obese patients, this publication will be justified. Here's my first question:

A person is looking for a highly competent obesity surgeon and is not sure about the best way to select one. Calls your office and requests a list of ten cases you operated upon so he/she can question those people about their experience with you, your team, and satisfaction with the hospital.

How do you react to that?

CARRASQUILLA: Patients who are considering weight-loss surgery (*WLS*) are very interested not only in discussing the operation with us, but also contacting other patients who already had this kind of treatment. This is one of the reasons why we hold monthly seminars at our institute. On these occasions, they have the opportunity to address their concerns and ask as many questions as they wish.

We also keep a record of names and phone numbers of patients who had obesity surgery so new patients are able to contact them directly in a personal and confidential manner. This, of course, is done with the previously treated patient's authorization.

MAREMA: At U.S. Bariatrics, our multidisciplinary team is dedicated to the success of each and every patient, from the very first encounter. And considering our patients are not only our most fervent evangelists, but also the greatest source of referrals to the comprehensive bariatric services we provide, we welcome every opportunity of connecting them with possible future patients.

We encourage prospective patients to attend one of our support groups so they can establish their own connections at a variety of stages in their weight loss and health journey.

CHAPUNOFF: What percentage of patients you treat with WLS (weight-loss surgery) are able to keep their weight normal or near to normal five years after surgery?

MAREMA: Five years after WLS, about 65 percent of patients have attained or closely maintained their target weight. However, 95 percent have lost at least half of their excess weight and 85 percent have lost at least three-quarters of their excess weight. Success depends on their compliance with behavior modification techniques, psychotherapeutic counseling, physical activity, and nutritional regime that our team promotes as a lifelong basis for ensuring optimal health.

CARRASQUILLA: Our statistics show that the average weight loss of all patients at twelve months after surgery is 71 percent of the excess weight. And five years after surgery, 70 percent of all our patients are able to keep their weight at a normal, or nearly normal level.

There is no magic in this surgery. It is a tool to assist patients in behavior modification throughout the weight-loss process and beyond. Conventional methods designed to correct it carry a dismal 98 percent failure rate.

Patients need to be in a state of perpetual self-vigilance and comply with the regimen and recommendations given to them. Methods they previously used did not succeed. It is up to them to preserve the benefits that resulted from WLS. Of course, close monitoring and medical follow-up will take care of minor problems before they become major concerns.

CHAPUNOFF: Would you please make some reference to the American Society for Metabolic and Bariatric Surgery (ASMBS) and the Surgical Review Corporation (SRC) and the vital role they play in our society?

MAREMA: Guidelines for proficiency of surgeons for bariatric procedures can be found at the ASMBS Web site www.ASMBS.org. An offshoot of the ASMBS is the Surgical Review Corporation, a pioneering organization dedicated to pursuing surgical excellence. It was formed to promote the delivery of bariatric surgical care with the highest levels of efficacy, efficiency, and safety. This company exists to check the qualifications and quality of care being performed by centers and surgeons who apply to them for certification. Please note that many centers will not be applying because they choose not to for a variety of reasons.

Patients, health care professionals, or insurers should visit the Surgical Review Corporation Web page to identify institutions and surgeons who are certified by this institution: www.surgicalreviewcorporation.org.

CHAPUNOFF: What about the training requirements for gastric bypass surgery versus the laparoscopic approach that just requires a few little "holes" in the abdomen?

MAREMA: The training requirements are different for open versus laparoscopic (lap) surgery. The lap requirements are more stringent than the open procedure given that a surgeon must acquire additional skills to be able to perform lap surgery.

In our hands at U.S. Bariatric, the lap technique is a safer approach than the open procedure due to less strain on the patients' body. Lap is also preferred by the majority of patients because of reduced pain and faster recovery.

The open Roux-en-Y gastric bypass operation (RYGBP) has been performed for decades on nonobese patients such as in the case of complicated ulcer disease. Thus, no special surgical training is needed to perform this procedure in obese patients.

The lap skills required to perform lap bypass and other bariatric procedures are being taught in lap fellowships throughout the United States. More importantly, greater than 50 percent of the training of Lap Surgical Fellows includes bariatric surgery.

CARRASQUILLA: The 1990s witnessed the pioneering work of a surgeon in Southern California, Dr. Alan Wittgrove, who had the audacity to perform the first gastric bypass operations using the laparoscopic technique.

The results were successful. He was instrumental in the development of what I shall refer to as the expansion era of obesity surgery. At that time, there were very few qualified surgeons doing WLS. From then on, the expansion of the technique mushroomed because of its excellent results.

Until recently, the training for the surgeon resulted from his/her individual experience, which made him/her responsible for his/her own education, and there was no organized collection of outcomes. The American Society of Metabolic and Bariatric Surgery decided to appoint a group of surgeons to form the Surgical Review Corporation for quality control and proceed with the selection of surgeons and centers that produce superior results.

What distinguishes a superior bariatric program from a mediocre one is not just the surgery itself, but rather the entire structure, from the selection of the patient to the postsurgical monitoring, patient education, office and hospital personnel, physical equipment, and so forth, all of which contribute to the execution of a superior program.

Tragically, and to the detriment of bariatric patients, the field has become contaminated by financial influences and is plagued with health insurance problems.

There is no board certification approved as yet for bariatric surgery, and the only parameters that we dispose of to categorize the center is a certification with a Center of Excellence by the Surgical Review Corporation, the peers and community opinions, and the dedication of the program.

CHAPUNOFF: I often see morbidly obese patients who have very little information about this disease and its surgical management. I have also noted that some health care providers frequently advise against obesity surgery when their own experience on the subject is nearly zero.

Would you comment on that?

MAREMA: Much of the negative physician response surrounding weight-loss surgery comes from what I like to refer to as the dark days when few doctors performed these operations.

A lot has been learned and improved over the fifty years that these operations have existed. Today, when health care practitioners position bariatric surgery in a negative light, they do so as an anecdotal response.

CARRASQUILLA: It is true that many people and some health care providers do not have enough information on the surgical treatment of morbid obesity. Preconceived notions prevail. This is not only sad but unfair as it results in unnecessary suffering and loss of life.

There are patients who have seen poor surgical results in friends or relatives. Although complications may occur—and do occur—at the best medical centers, generally speaking, their prevalence and gravity are greatly dependent upon professional knowledge, experience, and expediency.

Many doctors have an outdated knowledge and are not familiar with the existing state-of-the-art procedures that produce outstanding results. This lack of familiarity with the subject instills fear. It's a natural reaction: the typical fear of the unknown.

The current yearly death toll in the United States for obesity and comorbidities is approximately four hundred thousand patients, or about 1,100 people a day. It is incumbent upon all of us to do whatever we can to reduce this frightening statistics.

Unfortunately, some physicians have a financial interest in the administration of the patient's health care, and they act irresponsibly when they deny the referral of their patients for weight-loss surgery or provide patients false and misguided information to avoid the cost of surgery, knowing that the conventional form of therapy will carry a failure rate of 98 percent.

How can the executives of some insurance companies, the health care specialists working for them, and some practicing physicians deny patients who are in danger of becoming disabled or die, their quality life improvement or their survival? What entitles these people to act that way? Are they playing God, or what?

We once had a patient who came to see us on continuous oxygen therapy, electric chair, and electric car because she couldn't walk due to her obesity. She had been denied a referral to a bariatric surgeon by her primary care physician but obtained one with a new physician. Her former doctor told her to prepare to die. She had WLS with us, and now she is playing tennis with her daughter who also happens to be our patient.

CHAPUNOFF: I'm sure both of you could write a book just on those experiences! Let me ask you the next question, What kinds of gastrointestinal disorders present an absolute contraindication for obesity surgery?

CARRASQUILLA: In my opinion, surgery is contraindicated for obesity when the patient has active inflammatory bowel disease, active malignancy, and advanced liver cirrhosis. In any event, the surgeon must make a decision not based upon generalities but each individual case. Consultations with gastroenterologist and other specialists are helpful and necessary to reach a consensus about the best possible treatment for a particular patient.

MAREMA: Very few absolute contraindications to obesity surgery exist. Newly diagnosed cancers need to be evaluated on an individual basis for their impact on the patient's survival and for the ability of the body to fight disease if weight-loss surgery is performed. Some intestinal diseases, such inflammatory bowel disease, may impact the choice of operation.

CHAPUNOFF: What are the immediate or delayed possible postoperative complications that preoccupy you the most?

MAREMA: Failure to properly heal an area where the stomach or intestine was cut, stapled, or sewn, causing the juices that belong inside the intestines to leak into the abdomen and blood clots to the lungs, are the most worrisome immediate postoperative complications.

To prevent leaks, we reinforce the new stomach staple lines. In experienced hands, the risk of leak should be low.

We take special measures to prevent clots to the lungs, encouraging patients to resume walking the day of the surgery. The liberal use of blood thinners at the time of hospital stay is another layer of protection. Leg pumps during and after surgery further decrease the risks of clots forming.

It is interesting to note that blood clots in laparoscopic patients are extremely rare in comparison to the days when we performed all surgeries with the open technique (a long abdominal incision).

Delayed complications such as vitamin and mineral deficiency are worrisome. However, patients can easily prevent this by taking the recommended daily doses of bariatric supplements, specifically created for bariatric patients.

There is no reason today, with all the information available to bariatric professionals and bariatric patients for this to go undetected and untreated for any significant length of time.

CARRASQUILLA: As you know, major surgery predisposes to clot formation in legs, even in young healthy patients with normal body weights. This tendency is enhanced in obese patients.

If a venous clot turns loose and reaches the lung, it can cause trouble. It is the so-called *pulmonary embolus*. We try to prevent the formation of these clots by promoting active movements of the patient's lower extremities as soon as possible following surgery and also with special intermittent compression boots and blood thinners (anticoagulants).

An ever-present concern is the *leak*. This is a disruption of the wall of the pouch or the intestine, which could be serious enough to cause death if it is not discovered on time and treated effectively. There are other complications of relatively minor importance that occur in the context of any major surgical procedures.

As far as the patient is concerned, his/her most difficult moment, I believe, is the first postoperative day. This is the time when the patient wakes up from anesthesia and suffers some discomforts and begins to question his/her wisdom for having elected this kind of treatment. By the second day, he/she is feeling substantially better and is happy the worst is behind him/her.

CHAPUNOFF: Carlos, you introduced a new technique that substantially reduces the incidence of postoperative leaks. Can you tell us something about it?

CARRASQUILLA: The incidence of postoperative leaks is 2 percent to 5 percent. In our published one thousand cases we operated on, we only had one leak. Incidentally, the patient survived with medical management. A reoperation was not needed. So the results of our one thousand patients show a reduction of postoperative leaks down to 0.1 percent.

CHAPUNOFF: If your innovative method was widely used, what would that mean from the economic standpoint?

CARRASQUILLA: If we consider the total of 179,000 cases done last year only in the United States and if we estimate the average occurrence of postoperative leaks at 3.5 percent and if everyone using the technique I developed was equally successful—postoperative leaks down to 0.1 percent—about 1,880 lives would be saved annually. The calculator tells us that costs would be reduced by $1.2 billion a year.

Don't you think insurance companies would like the deal?

CHAPUNOFF: No, I think they'd love it. You'd be a kind of folk hero to them! Allow me to go back to the immediate postoperative gastric leak of the stomach contents through the suture line. You face two problems here:

1. Detection of the leakage, and
2. Decision about taking the patient back to the operating room

Leaking of stomach-intestinal juices leads to peritonitis. The diagnosis of peritonitis is particularly difficult in the morbidly obese. A person with normal weight will show a rigid abdominal wall, which will be obvious to the palpating hand of the examiner. This great diagnostic sign may be missing here. Sometimes, the leakage cannot even be confirmed by x-ray studies.

Can you tell me what goes on through your mind when you suspect a leakage, but you are not sure it's taking place. You must make a decision. You hate to take the patient back to the operating room. On the other hand, if you don't do that, the patient may not survive. How do you handle that?

MAREMA: Ed, the decision to return to the operating room is never easy. However, it should be stated that a return to surgery when the leakage is in doubt but it is suspected, is much better than an extended delay in reoperation that can lead to worse complications.

If a patient's vital signs are unstable after surgery and other causes of this instability, such as clots in the lungs are ruled out, then return is mandated.

Despite the difficulty in identifying clear signs that make the decision to return to surgery easy, a high index of suspicion and a willingness to proceed based on instinct must be part of the surgeon's armamentarium.

CARRASQUILLA: Recognizing the existence of a problem in the immediate postoperative period is extraordinarily important. I can't emphasize enough how important that is. And here, I must tell you, knowledge and experience really count. Incidentally, a persistent tachycardia (fast heart rate) always makes me suspicious of a possible leak.

CHAPUNOFF: There are a number of operations for obesity, and obviously, you always select one for a particular patient. What's your favorite procedure, and can you tell me why?

CARRASQUILLA: The preferred surgery nowadays is the Roux-en-Y gastric bypass (RYGBP). Besides the fast weight loss, patients with type 2 diabetes dramatically drop their blood sugar levels to the point where medications are often no longer necessary. A similar response is observed in hypertensive individuals. It's amazing to see how the blood pressure and the blood sugar improve so much, so quickly.

The most common operation performed in the world today for morbid obesity is the gastric bypass. The adjustable gastric band is a less-invasive procedure. We individualize the decision, and the choice of the method to be deployed is customized for each patient. I discuss all the details with the patient so he/she can participate in the decision-making process.

MAREMA: The Roux-en-Y gastric bypass (RYGBP) has been the gold standard of bariatric procedures for many decades. I love the technical challenges of this operation and the desire to perform it as flawlessly as humanly possible.

The adjustable gastric band is a safer operation, but patients lose weight at a slower pace and with less predictability than with RYGBP. There is much less to performing the adjustable gastric band from a technical standpoint.

However, I prefer to let my patients decide, in conjunction with advice from us, which procedures they would like to undergo.

CHAPUNOFF: Can you mention instances where you had to reverse a procedure and proceed to perform another one more suitable for that particular patient?

MAREMA: Revision of restrictive operations such as stomach stapling to a RYGBP is the most common of these procedures. It is mostly done in a patient with poor weight loss or due to problematic vomiting from the original surgery, being too tight. These operations fall in the category of revision operations and should only be performed by a surgeon who has demonstrated significant experience in primary bariatric procedures and has had special experience or training in the field of revisions as well.

CARRASQUILLA: That's right! And there have also been occasions when we had to reoperate on patients who had been treated at other facilities, who had had gastric stapling or small bowel bypass. We took them back to surgery and performed a Roux-en Y, which we considered it was a much better operation for those patients at those particular times.

CHAPUNOFF: What do you think about removing the gallbladder—cholecystectomy—at the time of gastric bypass surgery. This used to be done frequently in the past. In fact, I understand that some insurance companies demanded the removal of the gallbladder at the time of the weight-loss surgery, so two birds would be killed with one shot.

Rapid weight loss following successful weight-loss surgery is known to cause increased incidence of gallstones, so many surgeons used to remove the gallbladder during WLS to prevent future problems with stones. Can you tell us if you remove the gallbladder, or leave it where it belongs?

MAREMA: Presently, we do not perform gallbladder removal just because gallstones are found. Studies have shown that gallbladder removal is more risky when combined with RYGBP.

In our hands, less than 2 percent of patients with gallstones require gallbladder removal after RYGBP. Therefore, about ninety-eight out of one hundred of our patients do not need this operation, or conversely, we would have removed ninety-eight out of one hundred gallbladders that did not need to come out.

CARRASQUILLA: When we first started doing the gastric bypass, we used to remove the gallbladder as part of our routine. As time went by and more statistics became available, it became apparent that it was better not to touch a healthy gallbladder. This avoids subjecting the patient to the possibility of complications occurring from a secondary surgical procedure.

The incidence of gallbladder problems after gastric bypass proved not to be as frequent as it was believed years ago.

CHAPUNOFF: Nutritional complications post-gastric bypass procedures can be significant and also dangerous unless they are timely detected and treated expediently: deficiency of protein, iron, calcium, magnesium, potassium.

In your regular practice and in reference to this particular issue, do you prefer to follow the patient yourself at your institute or recommend the primary care physician to take charge of that responsibility?

MAREMA: We follow our patients for macronutrient (protein, fat) and micronutrient (vitamins and minerals) repletion in order to prevent deficiencies. These requirements, dosing, chemical compositions and monitoring are all defined specifically for bariatric patients. Nonetheless, we are eager to assist our patients' primary care physicians in managing these supplementations if they to choose, particularly if our patients are from out of town or move away from our centers in Fort Lauderdale and Orlando.

CARRASQUILLA: We have a routine on this: we like to follow our patients closely. Nutritional complications occur—and can be serious—when the patient does not follow the instructions given to him/her during the preoperative education.

CHAPUNOFF: I once saw a gentleman who had gastric bypass by one of you.

He weighed about six hundred pounds. It is one thing for a surgeon to get inside a patient's slim abdomen and quite another to reach the gut of a person who has extraordinarily thick adiposity.

An open abdominal incision gives you more exposure. Getting through the dense abdominal layers of fatty tissue is a tough proposition, a difficult job. Now when I see a few little holes in the abdominal wall that you use to do laparoscopic surgery, I wonder how you can get to the stomach and small bowel, do resections, and sew gastrointestinal tissues that are surrounded by a desperately abundant amount of fatty tissue. If you allow me plain speaking, this appears to me as difficult as hell.

MAREMA: Ed, lap surgery is technically challenging. There should be no mistake about that. The larger the patient, the more difficult it can be. However, lap surgery allows greater visibility and magnification of tissue planes and structures than open surgery in the larger patients. With experience, tactile stimuli are easily replaced by other means of assessing tissue planes and identification of vital structures, allowing us to successfully complete the operations. Experience is not to be underestimated.

CARRASQUILLA: At first glance, it would seem that an open abdominal incision would give you more exposure. However, with the scope and camera, you are able to see remote areas that are usually hidden to the naked eye. Of course, it is imperative that the surgeon be well trained and experienced to perform this surgery in this manner. We feel that laparoscopic surgery gives the patient the most favorable outcome.

The scope is a long, thin, tubular extension of the camera's lens and also carries the light into the abdomen with a fiber-optic system. As extension of our fingers, we use a long, very thin instrument, which allows us to dissect, cut, and suture. We also use a staple system, which produces very small staples that replace traditional sutures. Lately, the technology has advanced considerably and notably facilitates the performance of these procedures.

CHAPUNOFF: Bariatric surgery is being increasingly used in children. Do you have any comments on this?

CARRASQUILLA: I defer the treatment of children to pediatric bariatric surgeons. There are only a few experts on this field in the country. Unfortunately, there has been a considerable increase in the prevalence of morbid obesity in children too. Sometimes, obesity-related health problems affect kids before they reach adulthood.

MAREMA: It is essential to treat and prevent this pandemic increase in morbid obesity in children. In our experience, bariatric surgery is lifesaving in morbidly obese children who are mature and compliant. But don't mistake this for an endorsement of widespread application of surgery for children. These children, or rather adolescents, require extremely careful selection and close follow-up, often best done at children's hospitals or in the context of a very complete multidisciplinary program.

CHAPUNOFF: How many bariatric surgical procedures do you think a surgeon must perform to be considered by his peers to be a competent surgeon in the field. I'm talking about the kind of surgeon who you'd like to operate, let's say, on your wife, your daughter, your parents, or yourself?

MAREMA: I think this is two different questions. For lap bariatric surgery competence, about 100 to 140 cases is a safe number. This is a standard number of cases discussed among bariatric surgeons. As experience increases beyond these numbers, safety and success of the operation continue to improve.

When asking for me to select a caregiver for my family in this specialty, I am much more comfortable when the surgeon has performed at least five hundred or more procedures. There is a distinct advantage to the increased experience. Those surgeons who have that much experience understand this better than anyone else.

CARRASQUILLA: Ed, I believe more in competence and talent than in numbers. I consider that the number of performed surgeries is not as important as their outcomes. There has always been a first patient as well as the first one hundred patients.

It has been reported that the incidence of complications decreases after the performance of the first fifty cases, but I think this is very difficult to measure because the ability and dedication of the surgeon are of utmost importance. Nevertheless, other factors being equal; it's clear that the more training exposure and experience the surgeon gets, the more favorable will be the results.

CHAPUNOFF: I find it interesting that despite of the fact that your answer and Bob's are not similar, both of them make a lot of sense.

Let me shift my next question toward a more psychologically and behaviorally oriented area. Would you please share with me unusual sexual experiences of some of your severely obese patients? Certain aspects of the sexuality of these patients seem rather extraordinary.

I had a recent experience with a thirty-eight-year-old gentleman who was going to have WLS by one of you. He weighed 380 pounds and up to the point when his weight was three hundred pounds; he could have sex with his wife, *but only in the swimming pool.* He felt much lighter immersed in water and could perform fairly well. When his weight got over the three hundred pounds mark, his fatigue, shortness of breath, and the difficulties to find his penis hidden under his exceedingly prominent abdominal fat made it impossible for him to have sex.

Bob, do some of these experiences come to mind right now?

MAREMA: Yes, Ed, they do! There's one I couldn't forget even if I wanted to. The most bizarre event occurred at a support group when one of my patients approached me with the news that she had left her husband that day to pursue a relationship with me since I had done so much to change the direction of her life. I promptly explained that this was not possible and that she should return to her husband and seek counseling, both individual, and as a couple.

CHAPUNOFF: What a remarkable story that is, Bob!

MAREMA: Yes, Ed, it is. The psychological-emotional problems of the morbidly obese are rather peculiar. Obesity is an eating disorder, and those who suffer from eating disorders may, at times, swing from one extreme to the other. I once had a sexually abused patient who refused to eat years after gastric bypass surgery. She became thin and malnourished. In other words, she became anorexic. A few patients after bariatric surgery become averse to eating and become severely malnourished. The bottom line here is as follows: both overeating and anorexia may have underlying psychoemotional causes that have not been addressed by psychotherapeutic counseling applying behavior modification and cognitive therapies.

Unfortunately, a few of the patients who have gained weight after WLS professed envy of these thin malnourished patients, not realizing that both overeating and anorexia are unresolved manifestations of psychoemotional issues.

We occasionally see patients who are unable to eat post-WLS due transference of food addiction to alcohol abuse.

Rarely, we see patients who have successfully lost weight after WLS who are still very unhappy. They often trust that the first plastic surgery procedure to remove the excess skin in the abdomen, thigh, and arm will bring the very sought-after happiness. Months later and still unhappy, they hope and pray that cosmetic face surgery will finally bring them joy and peace of mind.

Some spouses feel threatened by the new attractiveness of their loved ones as they lose weight.

There's an increased incidence of sexual abuse in severely obese women. Thus, the strong need for psychotherapeutic intervention, counseling, and healing.

I've seen patients who developed substitution of food addiction by sex addiction, seeking extramarital relationships.

Male spouses of successful weight-loss partners often express how much they love the new body of their partner, and sometimes, they feel they have a new wife, or that they are actually cheating, having intimacy with another person.

Obese patients tend to be infertile and have decreased libido (sexual desire). As they lose weight, fertility is increased almost immediately. Nevertheless, they need to wait twelve to eighteen months after RYGBP surgery before considering and planning for pregnancy.

CHAPUNOFF: Carlos, I'm sure that you, like Bob, have learned about some patients' unusual intimate life experiences.

CARRASQUILLA: Yes, Ed, I have. Sometime ago, we operated on a gentleman who was just short of six hundred pounds. He had to depend on his mother for personal hygiene as he was unable to reach his genital area. In fact, he could never see his penis or even reach it with his hands to urinate. As a result, he would wet himself, and his urine would drip through his legs down to his feet.

He was extremely distressed, as one can expect. One year after his surgery, his weight came down 324 pounds. But he truly discovered "a new life" for his daily needs and activities when his weight dropped to two hundred pounds. His repressed sexuality also experienced a dramatic change. He wanted to catch up with his past sexual restrictions and became involved in multiple sexual encounters. In the process, he got hooked on drugs. He was being followed and counseled by a psychotherapist during all this period. Nevertheless, that wasn't enough to prevent him from getting into more trouble and was finally arrested.

The good news is that he ultimately recovered and is having a normal relationship with one woman. We are currently planning to operate another member of his family.

We also had a female patient who badly needed weight-loss surgery. Her husband decided against the operation out of fear that "she would become so beautiful that she might decide to leave him." He didn't want to take any chances!

CHAPUNOFF: The insecure husband you just mentioned reminds me of a forty-year-old lady who had gastric bypass. One year and a half later, she came to my office for a routine follow-up. She looked stunning, absolutely beautiful. And she was also very happy about her new life. Her husband couldn't take her success and sue her for divorce, which she gladly accepted.

He had abused her emotionally and psychologically during fifteen years of marriage. Her self-esteem was too low to react to her husband's behavior. He would always put her down, and he enjoyed being the dictatorial boss and having control of her. When she was transformed by WLS, her husband became insecure and increased his aggressiveness toward her. But she was a different person now and wasn't willing to tolerate his dominant role. He couldn't tolerate an assertive wife who had recovered her self-esteem. He needed someone he could step on, but he could no longer do that. So a divorce settled the discrepancies. By the way, the above interpretation was provided by a psychotherapist.

MAREMA: These and so many other experiences clearly show how strong the emotional-psychological components that accompany the morbid obesity condition are.

CARRASQUILLA: That's right! Unquestionably, the dynamics of patient-spouse, patient-relatives, patient-acquaintances changes after obesity surgery. Each case is different, of course, and poses different and specific challenges.

Fortunately, we also have patients who feel that WLS gave them a new life in every respect, socially, personally, physically, mentally, emotionally, sexually, and professionally.

CHAPUNOFF: How morbidly obese patients manage to have sex?

MAREMA: Actually, they seldom complain of this. The most frequently expressed problem is the difficulty in finding a mate. However, routine activities of daily living, such as personal hygiene, are sometimes problematic and may play a role in desire or either partner.

CARRASQUILLA: Males patients who normalize their weights enjoy very much, being able to see and touch their genitals after years of absence.

CHAPUNOFF: Carlos and Bob, we are at the end of this chapter, but we'll resume our conversation in the next pages dealing with patients' health insurance problems. I want to express my deepest gratitude to both of you for sharing your expertise with me and the readers.

CARRASQUILLA: Ed, I enjoyed this conversation very much. I thank you for the invitation to participate in your work.

MAREMA: I thank you too!

CHAPUNOFF: You're both most welcome!

CHAPTER 11

GASTRIC BYPASS SURGERY THE SURGICAL KNIFE COMPETING WITH PILLS AND INSULIN SHOTS IN THE MANAGEMENT OF DIABETES

Scientific discoveries sometimes result from unexpected observations, not because of preconceived planning.

The treatment of diabetes for the past half a century has been based on the same principles: diet, weight loss, oral medications, and insulin. New hypoglycemic drugs and new insulins—lente, semilente, ultralente—insulin pump have contributed to the management of the disease. But these therapies, at best, control the disorder. They don't make it go away.

Diabetes reduces life expectancy by an average of seven years. The complications of the disease may cause considerable grief and suffering: blindness, neuropathy, kidney failure, widespread vascular disease, wound infections, gangrene, amputations, heart disease, strokes, sexual dysfunction, among others, including a premature death. In fact, 70 percent of patients with diabetes still die prematurely from heart disease. The disorder is chronic and progressive and affects nearly twenty-one million Americans.

Many affected persons are young, so there are a number of personal as well as financial issues at stake.

It is an established fact that the control of the blood glucose levels minimizes complications and reduce mortality.

The American Diabetes Association (ADA) recommends treating most patients with diabetes to a targeted HgA1c of less than 7 percent.

In the early 1980s, it was observed that gastric bypass quickly dropped the blood sugar levels. In the past several years, the widespread use of gastric bypass operations for morbid obesity confirmed the fact that, yes, the glucose levels after bariatric surgery not only drop drastically, but do it in a few days, a couple of weeks, or one month *before any significant weight loss has occurred*. It was further observed that over 80 percent of morbidly obese patients who underwent gastric bypass surgery had total remission of the disease and no need for pills or insulin. This has been observed in dozens of studies involving thousands of patients.

This led to many believers to announce that a "cure" for diabetes has been found. Some diabetes experts are understandably concerned about this term and what it really means. To begin with, extensive and well-controlled studies are necessary to understand why the blood sugar drops so much soon after weight-loss surgery and also determine for how long patients will enjoy normal glucose levels. When the word "cure" is used, that implies that diabetes has disappeared, totally and permanently. Since patients need to be followed up for many years, nobody currently knows if the diabetes has been cured. Time (and research) will tell.

Although the excitement about the normalization of glucose levels following BS is fully justified and the phenomenon shows extraordinary promise, it seems more adequate to avoid the term "cure" until the fact is scientifically proven. Perhaps it would be preferable to call this phenomenon a "remission" or "regression" of diabetes.

Australian researchers reported that patients who had surgery to reduce the size of their stomachs were five times more likely to see their diabetes disappear over the next two years. The study's lead author, Dr. John Dixon of Monash University, Melbourne, Australia, feels that "it's the best therapy for diabetes that we have today, and it's very low risk."

Francesco Rubino, an Italian surgeon, conducted a series of experiments in diabetic rats. When he bypassed parts of their upper intestines, leaving their stomachs intact, the animals' diabetes disappeared. Dr. Rubino moved to New York Presbyterian Hospital/Weill Cornell Medical

Center to open a diabetes surgery center. He's also conducting a study, comparing standard treatment of diabetes with the treatment of diabetes by bariatric surgery.

The cure of diabetes is one of the dreams of the twenty-first century. And rightly so! Can you imagine what it means to prevent the disorders we mentioned above?

HOW DOES BARIATRIC SURGERY AFFECT THE BLOOD SUGAR

Restrictive operations such as the gastroplasties (adjustable band, vertical band, sleeve gastrectomy) reduce blood sugar levels by reducing food intake and also delaying the emptying of the stomach. GBP and BPD are both restrictive and malabsorption procedures. It has been postulated that these possibly act by changing the dynamics of gastrointestinal hormones secretion.

Bypassing the duodenum and the proximal jejunum probably decreases the production of a hormone that is responsible for the impaired action of insulin. It seems that the reduction of that hormone reclaims insulin's normal function and sensitivity, and the blood sugar levels come down.

This remarkable phenomenon has nothing to do with a decrease in food intake or weight reduction.

In different countries, there are studies in progress to learn what the gastric bypass does to the diabetes of the morbidly obese and also to the diabetes of patients who are just overweight. And there are also ongoing projects to evaluate the results of gastric bypass surgery in patients with type 2 diabetes who have a normal weight. This is just speculative at this time.

It would certainly be ironic that a little piece of metal, a surgical knife, turned out to be much more effective to deal with diabetes than all the traditional therapeutic methods used thus far. Can you imagine how the big pharmaceutical corporations' reaction would be if they ever found that the millions of dollars they spent over decades of hard work and research to produce drugs to lower the blood sugar levels were challenged by a surgically induced remission of diabetes?

Well, it's a bit too early to do that kind of projection.

If that proved to be correct and the precise mechanism by which the scalpel used in obesity surgery triggers the drop of the blood sugar becomes known, then the investigators' goal will be to discover a pill that will replace the blade.

CHAPTER 12

MISCONCEPTIONS, MISUNDERSTANDINGS, AND MISCALCULATIONS IN THE MANAGEMENT OF MORBID OBESITY

To err is human. The correction of errors is human too.

The American Association for Metabolic and Bariatric Surgery (ASMBS) estimated in 2006 that 177,600 people in the United States had bariatric surgery (BS) and that less than 1 percent of those who meet the criteria for surgery actually have surgery.

For a number of reasons that were detailed in other sections of this book, many morbidly obese patients do not qualify for weight-loss surgery (WLS)—some mental disorders, not enough motivation or willpower to comply with postoperative lifelong commitments, certain concomitant illnesses, and so forth. It is a different story when patients do indeed qualify for surgery, agree to have it, and for one unjustified reason or another, they are thrown out of the loop and do not have the operation.

The implications of such decisions are very serious and, at times, fatal. Disastrous outcomes for lack of timely and adequate treatment of morbid obesity are well-known. I'd like to offer some observations in this regard, hoping that they will lead to a better understanding of the reasons that explain these unfortunate situations.

1. THE PROFESSIONAL'S LACK OF FAMILIARITY WITH THE SUBJECT

The field of weight-loss surgery has recently made extraordinary advances. Many health care practitioners have not kept up with this information, and their opinions on the subject are based on what they knew or heard years ago when the field was evolving. They did not participate in the management of morbidly obese patients who were treated by first-class surgeons and are not familiar with the subject matter. This translates into hesitation and reluctance to recommend a radical treatment that will drastically change a person into another individual.

To recommend weight-loss surgery is a big deal. It is a serious decision. This is a major operation that may complicate with illnesses that did not exist prior to the operation, disability, or death. Although fatalities due to surgery are very infrequent, the idea may be intrusive and preoccupying to those who do not fully comprehend the whole picture and do not consider the enormous and far more frequent incidence of medical complications, including death, in those who are not treated the way they should.

Recommendations: A good point for health care practitioners to start the process of acquiring adequate information on morbid obesity and weight-loss surgery is to consult via Internet www.asmbs. org (American Society for Metabolic and Bariatric Surgery) and www. surgicalreviewcorporation.org (Surgical Review Corporation).

2. DOCTORS' ATTITUDE TOWARD HEALTH INSURANCE CORPORATIONS

- Accept the delays and postponements of the health insurance corporation without complaining about them the way they should.

If the patient is entitled to WLS, the doctor should be his/her advocate.

Note: I had several patients who were denied surgical benefits for their morbid obesity, and it took me less than ten minutes to call the medical director of the corporation and reverse a denial into an immediate acceptance by the insurance company to cover the cost of WLS. One of such cases happened recently. The patient had been wrestling with the insurance company for about one year without success. I requested to talk to the top medical executive of the corporation. He told me, "Doctor, your patient does not qualify for bariatric surgery." I replied, "Doctor, with all respect, I disagree with you 100 percent, and I'll tell you why." I did that. Then he said, "Your patient is being approved for coverage right now."

- There are health care practitioners who have contractual arrangements with HMOs, and they feel pressed to restrict the patients' access to the bariatric specialist because of economics. If they fail to comply with the restrictions imposed by the health insurance corporation, they could be neutralized and lose income.

Recommendations: Some doctors need to change their approach of detachment or indifference toward the morbidly obese who meet the qualifications to undergo WLS. They need to take a more determined and committed approach to speed up the process of insurance approval. Direct telephone calls to the medical director of health insurance corporations can be enlightening. It worked for me. I don't see why it wouldn't work for other physicians.

3. THE PATIENT'S INSUFFICIENT OR MISGUIDED INFORMATION

This is a very common problem. Many patients have no clear idea about the dangers of morbid obesity and how this disease can damage them. It is difficult for those concerned to make an informed decision when they haven't gotten the right information.

Recommendations: A person needs to learn more than "just a little" to understand morbid obesity's complications and what weight-loss surgery is all about.

I hope this book will help a little.

4. CORPORATE BEHAVIOR AND MISBEHAVIOR

I address this issue in chapter 13.

There are excellent American corporations that the patient and the doctor populations can work with without being hampered in their efforts to get bariatric surgery done when it is clear the patient's condition demands it.

There are others that are not so gracious and do whatever they can to avoid the coverage of WLS.

Recommendations: It seems to me that health insurance companies that are in the business of rejecting valid surgical cases of morbid obesity would be far more helpful to patients and themselves if they change their tactics and approve the approvable morbid obesity surgery cases sooner rather than later.

Changes in the law would help. I personally interviewed two Florida state senators, explained to them the unfairness of some insurance corporations to cover the costs of obesity surgery and the dreadful consequences that sometimes result from such behavior. They both agreed that "something should be done about that," but they never called me back.

The way I see it, some corporation and their executives expose themselves to legal action. A class suit involving patients who suffered disabilities or death from corporate negligence or mismanagement could run into the billions.

CHAPTER 13

MORBID OBESITY, THE INSURANCE COVERAGE ORDEAL, AND THE CORPORATE GREED SYNDROME

The treatment of morbid obesity demands action *instead of excuses, delays, procrastination, and rationalizations.*

The prestigious National Institutes of Health (NIH) set the *guidelines and criteria for qualification of weight-loss surgery*. You should be considered for obesity surgery if

- you have morbid obesity and have a BMI of forty or higher or a BMI of thirty-five associated with comorbidities such as hypertension, heart disease, sleep apnea, diabetes, degenerative joint disease (arthritis) of knees, hips, and lumbar spine;
- you had the condition for the past five years or longer;
- you have attempted, under a physician's care, other methods of weight loss for at least two years. These may include behavior modification, drug therapy, Overeaters Anonymous, Medifast, and/or other diets;
- no history of substance or alcohol abuse or complete recovery from them;
- you are psychologically apt to have such a drastic and permanent change in lifestyle, including, of course, your eating habits;
- you have realistic expectations and are fully aware of the risks and inconveniencies involved from having weight-loss surgery.

Let's first examine the basic steps that should be taken in order to attempt the approval by an insurance company to undergo WLS.

1. ROLES OF THE PATIENT

*   Read and understand your insurance company's "certificate of coverage." This can be provided to you by your employer or the insurance company.
*   Get a referral from your primary care physician. You need that support.
*   Keep detailed records of your efforts to lose weight, including weight-loss programs, diets, diet centers, fitness clubs, personal trainers.
*   Save receipts.
*   Document every visit to health care professionals for obesity-related issues.
*   Actively participate in the insurance preauthorization process.
*   Make personal phone calls to insurance companies.
*   If you are "technically" covered by an insurance company and the company refuses the coverage, you might need to obtain legal counseling.

2. ROLES OF THE PRIMARY CARE PHYSICIAN

He or she should do the following:

*   Write in his/her records all the existing comorbidities
*   List what kind of diet you used to lose weight
*   List medications used to achieve weight reduction
*   List medications you had to use because you did not achieve the desired weight loss
*   Note how many pounds you lost (or you didn't) with that diet
*   Write for how long you were able to keep your weight off and how long it took you to gain it back
*   Refer you to an obesity surgeon
*   Write a letter to your insurance provider recommending weight-loss surgery (WLS). This letter establishes the *medical necessity* of weight-loss surgery.

In that letter, he/she explains the following:

*   The medical reasons for the recommendation
*   Documents that previous attempts of the patient to lose weight by diet, drugs, and exercises have not produced results
*   Describes the conditions listed in guidelines and criteria (see above) that qualify you for surgical management of obesity

- If you have any significant gastrointestinal, liver, kidney disease, or any other significant physical ailments
- Results of thyroid tests
- Psychological, emotional, social, and economic consequences that are taking their toll, and that should be corrected to avoid future disability or death.

Note: If you meet the qualification points and your doctor is unresponsive to consider a consultation for possible WLS, consult another physician.

3. ROLE OF CONSULTING PHYSICIANS

It is important to present copies of various consultations reports by different specialists who were engaged in your case, documentation that morbid obesity contributed and was responsible for existing comorbidities. Examples are endocrinologist, if the patient has diabetes; rheumatologist or orthopedic for arthritis of hips, knees, ankles; neurosurgeon for lumbar (low back) disc disease; pulmonologist, if there's sleep apnea and treatment with CPAP machine or respiratory failure; cardiologist, for those who have disease of the coronary arteries or heart failure, etc.

4. ROLE OF THE BARIATRIC SURGEON

The bariatric surgeon writes a letter to the insurance company, detailing the indications for weight-reduction surgery.

5. FOLLOW-UP OF THE REQUEST FOR COVERAGE

- Call the insurance company in two weeks.
- If the request is denied, appeal the decision.
- If two weeks later the appeal is rejected, consider having an attorney sending the request.

6. YOUR ATTITUDE

You must be insistent and persistent. If it takes you one year to go back and forth with the insurance approval issue, take it!

If an employee of the insurance company gives you a hard time or appears insensitive to your requests or questions over the phone, don't be rude to him/her. Hang up and call again. Try another one. Don't create enemies.

7. At times, dramatic *steps need to be taken* to be covered by a health insurer, such as the following:

   * Changing jobs
   * Changing insurance provider
   * Changing doctors

INSURANCE COVERAGE

In most states of the union, legislation requires insurance companies to provide benefits for weight-loss surgery when patients meet the NIH criteria. (See page 147)

So technically speaking, the insurance coverage is widespread. In practice, the practical implementation of that coverage is often deficient. And it can be dangerous too. Delays in treating adequately morbid obesity may be responsible for disability and death.

Some insurers are very responsive and great to deal with. Others master the art of deception. A third category comes to terms with reality after testing the applicant's patience and endurance with excessive delays and repeated requests.

THE DISCRIMINATION QUESTION

Do some insurance companies have discriminatory attitudes toward the morbidly obese?

Standards applied by some insurance companies for the coverage of morbid obesity surgery appear to be different than those applied to other medico-surgical conditions.

It is standard practice to request authorization by medical offices and hospitals from insurance companies to proceed with all kinds of medical procedures and operations.

An orthopedic surgeon recommends a knee replacement, a general surgeon does the same for a bowel resection for colon cancer, a cardiologist balloons a coronary artery and implants a stent to prevent a myocardial infarction. There's objective of disease in all these cases. There's no problem with insurance coverage. *Why? Because these patients had (a) evidence of disease and (b) the need for the procedures.*

Now, *the morbidly obese has* evidence *of disease (morbid obesity itself is a disease), potentially disabling or life-threatening comorbidities and the need to undergo surgical correction in a short period of time, at times on urgent basis.* And yet quite often, he/she is subjected to excessive delays and appeals before their coverage is approved.

The attorney general of New York recently released a report that offers tips to consumers to obtain insurance coverage for obesity treatment.

"Obesity is a serious health issue," he said. "Health insurance plans often create obstacles to proper treatment." This report resulted from consumer complaints handled by the attorney general's health care help line.

Dr. Mitchell Roslin, chief of obesity surgery at Lenox Hill Hospital, New York, who was rated one of the top one hundred doctors by *New York Magazine* has said, "I think this is a slippery slope of discrimination. The surgery can be a matter of life and death, and if patients do not have surgery because they cannot afford to pay for it, the end result might mean death."

THE RATIONALE AND THE RATIONALIZATION ISSUES

A *rationale* is "an exposition of principles or reasons."

A *rationalization* is "the device of self-satisfying but incorrect reasons to satisfy one's behavior."

Some insurance corporations use a rationale and conveniently convert it into a rationalization.

Example: A patient carries 160 pounds of weight excess and had unsuccessful attempts to lose weight through exercise, diets, and antiobesity drugs. He/she is advised to undergo bariatric surgery. An insurance company either disqualifies him/her for the operation or delays excessively the waiting period for coverage.

One of the rationales used to justify that attitude appears to be based on the notion that if a patient didn't try all kinds of conservative methods to reverse morbid obesity, he is not entitled to insurance coverage.

Now, follow that line of reasoning and apply the principle to those who developed lung cancer from smoking. According to that kind of logic, patients should be disallowed health insurance coverage for lung surgery, radiation, or chemotherapy because they didn't try to prevent cancer by quitting smoking many years prior.

Treatment for lung cancer is, in fact, approved even if the patient neglected himself/herself by smoking two packs of cigarettes for the past thirty-five years and up until one second prior to the beginning of his/her therapy.

What about those who ate for decades tons of fat-loaded hamburgers, fries, and ice cream neglected to treat high blood pressure and carried a sedentary lifestyle. When they check into a hospital with an acute myocardial infarction, are they denied coverage because of their past neglectful habits?

The answer is *no*!

Or you mean to tell me that if you go to a party and drink excessively and as a result you get dizzy, fall and fracture your hip, the insurance provider will deny the expenses of the hospitalization and the needed hip surgery?

You think like that, and alcoholics wouldn't qualify for the coverage of liver cirrhosis; those with colon diverticulitis would also be rejected because they ate peanuts one day before the attack of abdominal pain. Reflux esophagitis and heartburn wouldn't be covered because the patient ate spicy Mexican food during his or her vacation, and so forth.

You don't tell a patient with liver cirrhosis, "You are not going to receive surgical-medical treatment for this condition because you neglected to stop drinking years ago," or "You are not entitled to receive treatment for AIDS because you failed to use the right condom at the right time four years ago."

Nevertheless, morbidly obese patients are often told, "You are not covered for obesity surgery because you ate too much. You ate the wrong food and did not exercise enough for the past year, two years, or five years."

What is that? A penalty for not "doing the right thing"? If this argument is accepted, one must accept that every time a person neglects himself/herself and causes an illness, he or she is not entitled to insurance coverage.

If you accept the concept of "personal neglect" by the morbidly obese, the decision not to cover him/her is discriminatory because other people who suffer ailments resulting from personal neglect are covered by insurance.

If you accept morbid obesity as "a disease"—and you must do that because it has been scientifically recognized as such—then the patient is entitled to insurance coverage.

I mentioned the patient's "personal neglect" argument just to tell you that even under those circumstances—if you are willing to accept it—the patient should be covered for the reasons I just explained. But *who has the right to define as neglectful the attitude of a person who suffers from an eating disorder or a psychological dysfunction that is beyond his or her control?*

Is it so easily—or conveniently—forgotten that morbidly obese patients reach their weights due to a combination of multiple factors, physical or psychological, that require specific therapy? Are you going to blame a person who has suffered sexual abuse, severe chronic anxiety, a bipolar or obsessive-compulsive disorder, severe injuries that led to forced bed rest for many years, severe eating disorders, etc., because that person is unable to control his/her binges?

When a patient has a life-threatening medical condition, you go ahead and treat that condition without paying any attention to the patient's own contribution to his/her ailment.

If it wasn't for the fact that morbidly obese patients are candidates for disability and death, the attitude of some insurance corporations would be laughable. Imagine that you're drowning in the ocean and somebody watching you has a lifesaver, and while you're desperately trying to remain afloat, you're demanded to explain why you didn't take better swimming lessons before.

One has to conclude that economics is the *only* reason behind these corporate decisions.

Laws must be changed.

Up until recently, obesity wasn't even considered a disease. Currently, it is! Good! Now and for the sake of so many lives in danger, so many dreams and aspirations that are being put on hold, insurers should develop the art and science of compassion, fairness, and expediency.

A DANGEROUSLY DELAYED WAITING PERIOD

When you deal with a serious or critical medical issue, there's only one question and one decision to make. How is the patient's problem solved *right now*?

Good doctors do not wait when they must act. In fact, they are *demanded*—humanly, ethically, professionally, and legally—to provide urgent medical or surgical treatments to those who need them. In the United States, even hard-core criminals receive urgent treatment when necessary.

I badly wanted to have the opinions of my two expert guests on this extremely important issue. Let's see what they have to say.

CHAPUNOFF: Robert and Carlos, some insurance companies deny or delay coverage for patients who clearly need obesity surgery. The patient is often required to document previous attempts to correct his/her weight, including various diets, exercises, and medications.

Anyone who deals with morbidly obese patients knows too well that the vast majority of them will not achieve the needed weight loss, and often, after losing, let's say, sixty pounds, they will gain them back.

Unquestionably, not every morbidly obese person qualifies for WLS. Personality disorders, psychological and physical dysfunctions of various kinds disqualify certain patients for the procedure. But it is also beyond any question that many severely overweight patients badly need the operation, and a prolonged waiting period might end in disaster.

Those who need WLS are at risk of having a heart attack, heart failure, stroke, and a host of additional potentially disabling or lethal complications.

Some insurance corporations are excellent, but others seem to be far more interested in profits than the well-being of their clients.

Would you please share with us your thoughts on this issue?

CARRASQUILLA: Yes, Ed, I agree with you. I recently had a meeting with a couple of executives of a large insurance company (I'm not a provider for that company). I was told that they were in the business of eradicating a number of physicians from their programs and "compacting the network."

I naively asked them if the purpose of such changes aimed at improving the quality of the involved professionals. Their answer was shocking! They said, "We don't care about your medical outcomes and how successful the results of your operations are. When we review you, we check the billing, the costs. We want physicians who are cost-efficient, not better surgeons."

That ended the conversation. This insurance company I'm referring to hires people with little knowledge in charge of key departments and calls them managers of Network Systems or whatever. The bottom line is clear: this particular corporation is far more concerned about making money than worrying about the welfare of its clients.

I must also tell you that we also deal with great insurance companies that are concerned about the well-being of the patient population.

Those affected by morbid obesity have to "shop around" for the right insurance company, as much, and as carefully, as they do in the search for good doctors.

A patient of mine, an unfortunate gentleman who had been fighting his insurance company because of an exclusion for obesity in his contract finally found a solution.

Having no hope of getting assistance from his insurer, his family helped him financially, so he could proceed with the operation.

I saw him at my office on a Thursday. His medical condition was poor and needed bariatric surgery fast. We gave him a few days for his preoperative work up and had an appointment with us next Monday. He did not show up. Why? He expired during the sleep on Sunday. If you call this an unnecessary tragedy, you're correct!

CHAPUNOFF: Yes, Carlos, you're right! That is a tragedy! In some instances, patients who suffer from morbid obesity appear to be insured by companies that suffer from morbid greed!

Some years back, I had a similar experience with a cardiac patient for whom I had recommended cardiac transplantation. There are still times when I wake up in the middle of the night and see the sweet smile he had gifted me with for giving him a ray of hope. I can't leave that pain behind me!

Bob, would you tell us about your feelings and experience on this touchy affair?

MAREMA: Ed, I would characterize my relationship with insurance companies as a love-hate relationship. You love the fact that they give you a sense of security, in the sense that your needs will be met when the time arises. However, you hate the fact that when it is determined that the patient qualifies for obesity surgery, they often refuse to cooperate. That means, of course, that the necessary funding is not provided.

There is no question about the fact the morbid obesity is one of the leading causes of preventable deaths in the United States today. We operate very sick patients who badly need to get rid of their morbid obesity. Truly, there is no medical or scientific justification for denial of care. This is a pure economic issue.

In order to succeed in business, a company must make profit. When this is a publicly traded company, such as an insurance company, the greater the profit, the more secure the future of its executives is. Focus shifts from overall health of its members to quarterly profits. In order to hold on to their dollars, they constantly change the rules of the plans. This is often disguised by the offering of new coverage products that cause employers and benefits administrators to select an ever-decreasing array of services to a lesser cost.

There is irrefutable evidence in the medical literature as to the improved health, decreased risk of developing life-threatening illnesses, decreased risk of death, and overall improved quality of life for those patients who undergo weight-loss surgery. Yet many insurance companies characterize this surgery as unproven, experimental or worse, detrimental to their members as if they are doing their members a favor by preventing them from having surgery. Gastric bypass surgery is not a new operation. It has been around for the past fifty years, and new techniques make it safer and less traumatic.

My belief is that this insurance problem is just a manifestation of corporate greed cloaked in misinformation and represents another example of discrimination. This time, the discrimination is against the obese who are not vocal or activist-oriented group, thus it continues. If this was denial of care for cancer, maternal-child, heart disease, AIDS, or any other disease state, there would have already been a public outcry that would have shifted policy.

Obesity is a disease of epidemic proportions. Measures to deal with it must include not only medical or surgical therapeutic modalities, but also those aimed at prevention.

The voice of the morbidly obese is not heard today. There are legions of patients who wait in vain for an operation such as gastric bypass that would give them the gift of life and the control of coexistent medical illnesses that would return them to a normal life and prevent them from suffering strokes, diabetes, hypertension, renal, pulmonary and heart failure, and sudden death, among many other painful and disabling maladies.

The indifference of certain insurance corporations toward the suffering of the morbidly obese must end!

CHAPTER 14

A DECISION THAT CHANGED THE COURSE OF A LIFE . . . AND SEVERAL OTHERS

One practical experience is worth a thousand theoretical explanations.

From the time I began writing this book to the time it was nearly completed, I never expected to come up with this chapter. But then one evening, while working on this project and going over papers and more papers, I found photos that a patient had sent to me years prior plus a note she had written for me.

I had kept the photos and note because they possessed great spiritual value to me. I don't receive this kind of recognition in writing every day. But from time to time, I do, and I must admit, I enjoy the patient's gesture immensely.

I am not reporting this experience for personal advertisement. To begin with, what I did—namely, the recommendation to my consulting client to undergo obesity surgery—was a professional and ethical duty on my part. I do not hang medals on my chest for fulfilling my duties and obligations, or doing what I'm supposed to do.

So the real reason for writing this chapter about Mrs. Muniz is the potentially significant impact it may have on those who suffer from morbid obesity and qualify for weight-loss surgery and who are in the process of deciding what to do next.

A few lines below, you'll see her note and the photos she personally delivered to me on January 26, 2004.

This is the way it happened: Approximately three years ago, she was referred to me for a cardiology evaluation because she was having pains in her left arm while doing moderate physical exertions. She suffered from morbid obesity and a substantial number of obesity-associated illnesses.

That visit marked the beginning of a process that ended in her gastric bypass surgery. It wasn't an easy ride for the patient, but the results were highly gratifying.

Mrs. Muniz happens to be a courageous, motivated, and disciplined person. And she also has a beautiful natural quality—I'd call it generosity. Unquestionably, it is generous on her part to share details of her private life with all of us. She has been trying to convey to others the message of her own experience, the deep concern, pains, and vicissitudes she had to endure for so long, and what it means to have become almost as light as a feather.

Figure 33. June 2003—257 pounds   March 2006—125 pounds

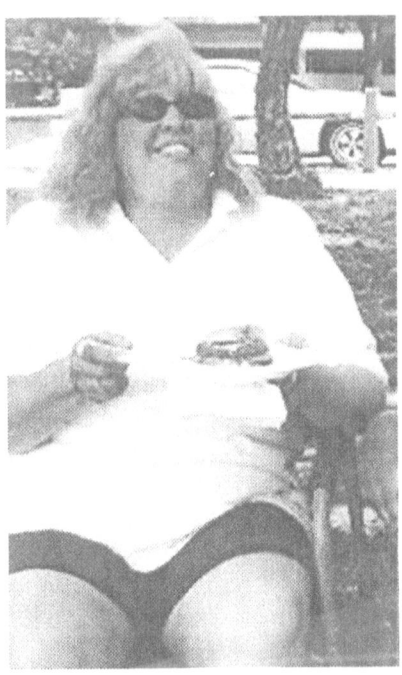 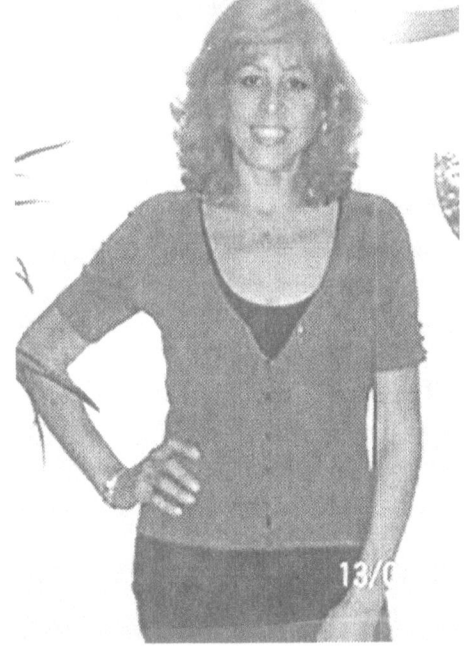

1/26/2004

Dear Dr. Chapunoff,

Here are the photos I promised you. My starting weight was 257 on June 9th, 2003. The recent photo is January 15th, 2004. I have lost 96 pounds so far, I have 20 pounds to go.

Thank you again for being the only doctor who agreed to the Bariaric surgery. I have my life back now, thanks to you!

Sincerely,

Ileana Muniz (signature)

Ileana Muniz

And now, let's see what Mrs. Muniz decided to share with us.

CHAPUNOFF: Ileana, first of all, let me thank you very, very much for your willingness to share your experience with me and the rest of the world, dealing with what used to be a nightmare for you that eventually turned into a wonderful reality.

ILEANA: Dr. Chapunoff, I also want to thank you for inviting me to tell my side of the story. I always try to help those who suffer from this condition. So many people are affected by morbid obesity! The trouble is that, for a number of reasons, legions of patients never get treated with weight-loss surgery. Passivity in approaching the treatment of this disease can cause disability and death, as you well know.

CHAPUNOFF: I agree with you, Ileana. Would you tell us about your own experience? Please go back to the very beginning. We do not have a psychotherapist monitoring our conversation and giving us expert psychological interpretations. So we'll have to do it our own way. I have no problems with that, and obviously, you feel the same way.

A significant number of morbidly obese patients have or have had some unpleasant emotional and situational encounters in their lives, and I'll first try to touch base with you on that particular issue.

According to the way *you* feel, what was the triggering factor that started the dysfunctional eating process?

ILEANA: When I was a child, I was sensitive to my mother's remarks about my physical appearance. Looking back to those days, I think her attitude toward me was detrimental. She was a beautician. That wasn't the problem though. The real problem was that she wanted me to be beautiful, very beautiful. She placed extraordinary emphasis on physical beauty and demanded from me to be physically "perfect."

This attitude created my self-image problem. No matter what I did to please her, she wouldn't be satisfied. She wanted more. I tried very hard. You know, a child tries to make her mother and father happy. I had no success with that. So I always thought that I was physically ugly.

When I see the photos taken at twelve years of age, retrospectively, I believe I was a pretty girl, but that's not the way I felt about myself then.

That, in my opinion, was the beginning of the eating disorder. An enormous sense of frustration and the anxiety that comes with it.

CHAPUNOFF: Did anything else of importance happen in your childhood that further aggravated your uncontrolled weight gain?

ILEANA: Oh yes! Definitely!

CHAPUNOFF: Could you tell us what it was?

ILEANA: Certainly! I was sexually molested on several occasions by two individuals when I was between five and nine: one was an uncle and the other a stranger.

CHAPUNOFF: Gee! That was really bad!

ILEANA: It sure was! It was devastating!

CHAPUNOFF: This is a touchy issue, but with your permission, and hoping I'm not abusing your kindness in any way, I'd like to ask you a question on these sexual incidents: What kind of psychological-emotional reactions did you have resulting from those experiences that lead you to consume large quantities of food?

ILEANA: Don't feel bad about asking me these questions, Dr. Chapunoff. I'm very comfortable talking to you about them, and I'm also happy to know that my traumas and unpleasant experiences will help others.

Getting to the question you just asked me, what went through my mind after the sexual molestation experiences? This is the way I reacted: I felt that I did not want to be pretty. In fact, I wanted to be ugly.

CHAPUNOFF: May I ask you why?

ILEANA: Yes, of course. I wanted to be ugly so no one would ever touch me again. I wanted to be rejected, undesired. That was purely a defensive posture, a shieldlike protection.

CHAPUNOFF: Ileana, do you remember your weight at age twelve?

ILEANA: I remember it well! 215 pounds. I had plenty of yo-yo fluctuations. At the age of sixteen, I weighed 140 pounds.

CHAPUNOFF: How was your social life during adolescence? Did you relate to other people?

ILEANA: Not really! I felt quite isolated. Up until the time I met my future husband at eighteen, I'd had no dating, no social life. We married when I was twenty.

I did something though that will surely call your attention: between age five and twenty-five, I studied dance and did regular exercises with it. As an attempt to make me more graceful, my mother insisted on ballet lessons, which later became a passion for me, to this day.

CHAPUNOFF: You're right! I didn't expect that kind of activity in your younger years when you had so much to deal with. What kind of dance did you do?

ILEANA: I did classical ballet and jazz.

CHAPUNOFF: You've been married for thirty-four years and had a son who now lives in California. I understand your husband Pete has always been very supportive.

ILEANA: Yes, that's true. Pete is a very special man. We have a successful marriage. He never made any comments about my physical appearance when I was severely overweight. His concerns were the possible consequences of morbid obesity on my general state of health. He's a tolerant, patient, and loving man.

CHAPUNOFF: I'm sure he is. I know he's currently an assistant principal at a junior high school. In our contemporary times, you've got to be a virtuous person to hold on to that position.

ILEANA: I don't disagree with that!

CHAPUNOFF: You're also a teacher, right?

ILEANA: Yes, I am. In addition, I'm the magnet coordinator of foreign languages.

CHAPUNOFF: Ileana, would you tell us how you've got involved *medically* with your condition. What prompted you to seek professional help?

ILEANA: My therapy journey, if I can call it that way, began in June 2002 at 260 pound and size 22. I was fifty and suffering asthma, sleep apnea, unexplained pain down my left arm, high blood pressure, skin rashes, urinary incontinence, osteoarthritis, double herniated spinal discs, depression, and shame.

I was at my wit's end with medications and the feeling that I was way too young to feel so old. I approached my family physician with the idea of bariatric surgery, but she discouraged it, saying that it was too drastic, and she thought I could take the weight off by myself with diet and exercise. Well, I had tried that . . . for forty years! And probably with every diet known and unknown to man.

I pursued bariatric surgery anyway. I went to U.S. Bariatric, Fort Lauderdale, Florida. There, I met Dr. Robert Marema. His expertise and talents preceded him.

I was recommended to see a cardiologist when I began feeling pain radiating down my left arm each time I tried to exercise, and I was referred to Dr. Eduardo Chapunoff.

CHAPUNOFF: That name sounds familiar. I think I know that guy!

ILEANA: Yes, I'm sure you do!

CHAPUNOFF: I certainly do remember we had the interview, but since I saw many patients since, I can't remember what I said to you during that consultation. You probably have a better recollection.

ILEANA: Oh sure, I clearly remember our conversation! You took one look at me and said something that changed my life forever. You said I would not live much longer to see my own grandchildren born unless I lose at least one hundred pounds. It hit me then! I was going to die! I went home and cried. I had to take action! I had a follow-up visit with you, and I told you about the surgery I wanted. You told me, "If your family physician does not agree to recommend you for obesity surgery, I will do all I can to sway your insurance carrier to approve you!"

Then my family physician changed her mind. So we decided to forge ahead, and I was approved immediately. I was scared, ecstatic, and excited. I underwent surgery on June 9, 2003.

It took less than a year to shed 120 pounds. My hair fell out; my skin lost all elasticity and hung in ugly folds all over my body. It was a bit scary for a while, but I hung in there. I tried to stay positive and deal with my lifestyle change. My hair eventually grew back in long and glossy, and I was mental about taking all my supplements and maintaining a good diet.

My asthma, sleep apnea, incontinence, arm pain, arthritis pain, disc pain, and high blood pressure completely resolved! I was off the CPAP and all medications at last! But I was becoming more and more depressed at the awful shape of my body and skin. I was determined to go on with the next step: plastic surgery.

This happened two years after my obesity surgery. I was keeping my weight down to 132 pounds, and I'd gotten into size 6. Never in my wildest dreams did I think this was possible. My new addiction was clothes shopping. Making up for the lost time and looking cute!

I had plastic surgery (a tummy tuck, a breast lift, and a torso contour) nine months ago.

Now it is almost three years out of bariatric surgery. I am at 125 pounds and a size 4. Actually, I took off an additional ten pounds I didn't expect, so I am a bit underweight for my height. Oh, booohooo!

CHAPUNOFF: Ileana, your candor and openness are greatly appreciated. Can you tell us something about the way you eat these days, how careful you are, your discomforts, and so forth?

ILEANA: I've learned to eat differently, of course. I had a Roux-en-Y procedure. I never eat a big meal. I never eat a normal size meal either. If I go to a restaurant, I only eat a fraction of the meal and take the rest home in a doggy bag. I must take my time to chew food. I cannot rush the swallowing of food. If I rush the process and eat fast, I have a very uncomfortable sensation in the lower part of my chest.

CHAPUNOFF: Do you ever eat something you are not supposed to?

ILEANA: Very infrequently!

CHAPUNOFF: And when you do, what happens?

ILEANA: When I yield to just one little bite of cake or a doughnut, I experience the dumping syndrome: palpitations, nausea, profuse perspiration. I still have times when I eat too fast and feel sick for up to an hour afterward.

CHAPUNOFF: Ileana, do you have any regrets about the bariatric surgery you had?

ILEANA: Yes, I definitely do! My only regret is not having had it sooner while I was younger. The more time I allowed to pass, the more devastation to my organs and skin, not to mention my psychological state.

I am a new woman, and I thank all my doctors and God for these blessings! All in all, this has been a wonderful, exhilarating journey. I have never been happier with my health and weight. Finally, I'm enjoying the life I was meant to live.

It is March 2006. I just had my fifty-fourth birthday. I have the body of a twenty-five-year old. Perhaps more significantly, I really feel twenty-five again!

CHAPTER 15

MORBID OBESITY AND BEHAVIOR THERAPY

A person's behavior decides his/her fate.

The eminent psychotherapist, Dr. Arnold A. Lazarus, who is currently distinguished professor emeritus of psychology at Rutgers University, was one of the pioneers of behavior therapy in the 1960s, and the world owes him plenty because of it.

One of his books titled *Multimodal Behavior Therapy* was published in 1976. A collaborator Dr. William L. Mulligan wrote chapter 14 and named it "A Multimodal Approach to the Treatment of Obesity." Many years have passed since, but the therapy principles described in that book continue to have extraordinary value.

The case of a woman who was treated with twenty-five individual sessions was described.

One of the therapy features that called my attention was the "contract" that therapist and patient agreed upon: she would call Dr. Mulligan—any time day or night—if she felt she was about to go off of her diet.

I don't know how often nowadays a therapist provides that kind of professional service to patients. There is a current trend to treat obese patients with group therapy rather than on one-to-one basis.

The therapy dealt first with the patient's eating behavior. She was trained in deep muscle relaxation, agreed to stop drinking since alcohol was incompatible with the Weight Watchers Diet she was following. She had less control with food on weekends, so she was instructed to find more constructive and enjoyable weekend activities. She was also told that she would have to change her eating habits on a permanent rather than on a temporary basis.

It was recommended that she (a) only eat when she was sitting at her kitchen table, (b) write down everything she planned to eat just before doing so, (c) place her silverware on the table after each mouthful, and (d) chew her food twenty-five to thirty times before swallowing.

These procedures were designed to slow down the rate at which food was ingested and to change eating from an automatic, habitual response to a set of specific behaviors over which the patient could gradually gain conscious control.

As you can appreciate, everything offered to the patient was designed to induce radical behavior modification.

The treatment produced a weight reduction from 210 pounds to 130 pounds.

The psychotherapist also explored and dealt with her affect and emotional problems, sensations (tension and anxiety), imagery (unrealistic image of herself as an obese woman), cognitions (malignant self-criticism, feelings of worthlessness), interpersonal relationships (intimate, social, family, etc.), drugs (medications prescribed by a psychiatrists were discontinued).

Half a century passed on since this effective therapeutic approach took place, and current therapists continue to use the same basic principles. And they are *good* principles.

If you ask me what we did in cardiology fifty years ago, I can only tell you that almost everything we do these days is different. We can only be grateful for that!

THE PRESENT TREND

Currently, most behavioral programs are offered in a group format with six months of weekly meetings followed by six months of biweekly meetings and six months of monthly meetings.

There is a multidisciplinary team of specialists trained in nutrition, exercise physiology, and clinical psychology. Structured series of lessons are designed to teach participants to modify their diet and exercise behaviors.

Self-monitoring is considered an essential aspect of the program.

Patients write every thing they eat, count calories, and review their records on food and physical activities with their therapist. They are instructed to reduce portions size, avoid unhealthy products and eat out at restaurants (if that's a source of temptation), only have low-calorie snacks in the house, and select friends and acquaintances who understand their problem and offer them support and understanding.

The psychotherapist also focuses on other problems, e.g., lack of support by close relatives and friends, poor exercise compliance.

BEHAVIORS THAT WILL HELP YOU LOSE WEIGHT AND MAINTAIN IT

1. **Set an acceptable and reasonable goal.**
   Make sure it is (a) specific, (b) attainable, and (c) forgiving (accept your own imperfections).

   a) Specific. Instead of saying, "I'm going to do more exercise," be specific and get ready for a real life number, let's say, walk for thirty minutes every day.
   b) Attainable. Suppose that you were correct about being specific and set a goal of walking thirty minutes every day. But you might have been wrong in setting the goal of exercising "every day." Perhaps it would be more attainable to say, "I'm going to walk five days a week." Make it a bit easier on yourself.
   c) Forgiving. Don't feel guilty because you are not killing yourself in your exercise program. You don't have to.

2. **Reward your success.**
   A little gift or special moment with your family such as one day or two at a vacation resort.
3. **Become efficient in self-monitoring.**
   Record what you eat, consumed calories, activities and exercises, the kind of physical activity you do and how much and how often you do it. Remember that *you* are in charge of your life, not your physician or psychotherapist. These professionals will offer you advice

and recommendations, but you'll be the one in charge of making decisions—how much you should eat, the time you should do it, what foods you should never look at.

4. **Be careful about the way you evaluate your weight changes.**
   Your body's water weight will change much more from day to day than your fat weight. Water changes don't mean anything in relation to your weight-reducing efforts.

5. **Control your environment.**
   Select an eating schedule that helps you to avoid skip meals or delay them. This might lead you to eat more later.

   Avoid having any kind of high-calorie foods at home.

   Be careful about inviting people at home for parties or attending those in other places.

With these approaches, the weight losses achieved in the most successful group averaged 10.5 kilograms at six months, 11.5 kilograms at twelve months, and 8.3 kilograms at eighteen months.

That's about the best that can be achieved in weight loss with behavior therapy.

Lifestyle Changes

Changes in physical activities should be implemented, including using stairs instead of elevators or avoiding "disability parking" in parking lots or getting off the bus one stop earlier or walking from store to store.

It is also important to select the type of exercise or physical activity that the person enjoys. This will increase the likelihood of compliance and long-term adherence.

How Much Exercise Is Advisable?

It's important to start slowly and gradually. Then the activity may be incremented by walking two miles a day five days each week.

The National Weight Control Registry participants lost more than sixty pounds and kept it off for longer than six years expending an average of 2,800 kilocalories per week.

This can be done by performing different activities such as dancing, walking, bicycling, or strength training.

Calories Losses for Ten Minutes of Physical Activity

Activity	Caloric expenditure
Walking (4 miles/hour)	72
Swimming	56
Dancing	48
Cycling (13 miles/hour)	124
Light gardening	42
Shoveling snow	89

Low Calorie versus Very Low Calorie (VLC) Diets

A low calorie diet contains 1,000-1,500 kilocalories per day. A VLC contains four hundred to eight hundred kilocalorie per day.

Long-term results do not justify the use of a VLC.

With these low-calorie diets, maximum weight loss is achieved in about six months. The trouble is that weight is regained. This is thought to be due to several reasons:

- Weight loss lowers metabolic rate and leptin levels. These changes promote weight regain
- Many patients never reached the preset target weight loss and become frustrated
- Boredom causes frequent failures

Who Has a Better Chance of Losing Weight?

Initial body weight is the most consistent pretreatment predictor of treatment outcome.

Heavier subjects achieve larger short-term and long-term losses.

Medical Status

Some medical conditions or events influence the course of behavior modification program.

- Cardiovascular disease (angina, heart failure, myocardial infarction), knees, feet, hip, or low back pain, uncontrolled hypertension, severe anemia, and a host of other ailments may disconnect the patient from his/her program.

- Some antidepressants, insulin, treatment with steroids, postquitting smoking weight gain make the weight-loss program much more difficult.
- Mental illnesses that are not well controlled by medications also offer increased resistance to weight loss (bipolar, obsessive-compulsive disorder, schizophrenia, anxiety, depression).
- Binge eaters tend to have a more complex psychopathology and are thought to achieve poorer result in weight-loss efforts compared with nonbinge eaters

The scientific approach to morbid obesity treatment with diets and psychotherapy is evolving. To achieve long-term success in the therapy of this condition, new modalities of treatment are needed.

CHAPTER 16

OBESITY AND EXERCISE: GET GOOD ADVICE ON THIS TOO: PREVENT INJURIES

Exercise is one of the most economical and accessible methods to treat obesity, and yet it is the most neglected.

It is true that morbid obesity is a complex disease, and its origins can be traced to genetic influence, psychological dysfunctions, hormonal imbalances, serious injuries with prolonged bed rest—sometimes during many years—and other factors. But it is also true that lack of exercise is an extremely frequent cause of obesity.

Many obese patients carry on lives with near total physical inactivity. Typically, they sit in front of a computer for ten hours a day then watch TV for two to three hours—if not more—and go to sleep. They adhere to this pattern for decades. For them, this becomes a way of life.

A person's weight is essentially the result of his/her food consumption and the expenditure of energy.

In the Western culture, a decline in physical activity characterizes both working and leisure-time pursuits. Machines have replaced most of man's physical efforts, including those used for entertainment, such as video games. Visual and audio senses and the motion of one-hand fingers have substituted the energetic pace of various sports. These rituals are practiced consistently for long periods of time and lead to the inexorable process of fatty tissue accumulation.

The prevalence of obesity and the proclivity to reduce physical activity also affect children and all levels of economic and racial groups.

Regular exercise would certainly contribute to improve currently gloomy statistics. It is estimated that approximately three hundred thousand adult persons die per year in the United States because of obesity. Sixty-four percent of American adults are overweight or obese (BMI of twenty-five kilograms/m$_2$ or higher).

Some of these demises are probably related to low fitness. It is a fact though that the heavier the weight, the more serious are the resulting medical complications.

Poor physical activity promotes obesity (due to little energy expenditure), and obesity promotes inactivity (due to exhaustion caused by minimal ambulation). So it is a vicious circle, a self-perpetuating phenomenon.

Recent data indicates that 28.7 percent of adults in the United States participate in *no* physical activity and 45.9 percent do so little that could never derive any benefits from it.

It is clear that in order to *achieve and maintain* a normal weight, three basic elements are required:

- Adequate physical activity
- Diet
- Behavior modification

Adequate physical activity. Every person enjoys certain physical activities and dislikes others. The selection will depend upon your personal taste and your physical limitations. Examples: You like to walk, but severe knee, low back, hip or foot pain makes ambulation difficult, or you enjoy yard work but live in a condo apartment where there's no grass to cut, or you like pool exercises but have no pool at your disposal, or you'd love to try double tennis, golf, or biking, but your weight has already gone too far for you to do these things. Fatigue, shortness of breath, or arthritic pains won't let you do it!

Diet. Humans, we all know, are far from perfect, and mistakes are made in any weight-reducing program due to temptations, omissions, and neglect. Yet substantial weight loss is possible as long as the imperfections are minimal, infrequent, and corrected on time.

Radical behavior modification. To be effective, it must be permanent.

WEIGHT LOSS AND EXERCISE

A physical activity program can result in significant weight loss but only if the amount of exercise is substantial. The start should be slow and with gradual increments.

The goal of exercise is not only to achieve weight loss, but maintain that loss. Helpful activities include walking, stationary or road cycling, treadmill, aerobics, hiking, weight lifting, stair stepping.

To maintain weight loss, sedentary individuals would have to add eighty minutes per day of moderate activity, such as brisk walking, or thirty-five minutes of vigorous activity, such as fast cycling or aerobics.

Those who sit for long hours at their jobs should cut down their sitting time and do brisk walking every hour for three to four minutes.

Studies have shown that improving fitness had a greater impact on mortality risk than losing weight. Data indicates that overweight and obese individuals who are physically active and fit have a lower risk of morbidity and mortality than normal-weight individuals who are sedentary and unfit.

Compliance with a regular program of exercises gives you more energy and a healthier life. You'll have more stamina, relieve part of the stress and anxiety, improve your balance, coordination, and flexibility. It'll also gift you with a more positive attitude.

OBESITY AND MEDICAL COUNSELING

At least 50 percent of obese patients do not receive exercise counseling from their physicians.

Only 20 percent of patients are ready to follow a program of exercise when prescribed by a health care professional.

Most patients who receive counseling on physical activity show poor adherence to those programs.

It's been observed that thirty minutes daily of regular, continuous physical exercise has the same effect as five to fifteen minutes of periods of activities spread throughout the day as far as weight control and cardiorespiratory fitness.

Sometimes, strict adherence to medical recommendations is not followed. The patient was advised exercises thirty minutes a day, seven days a week, but he/she is willing to do them for twenty minutes a day, five days a week. The professional must be flexible and understanding.

FREQUENT OBSTACLES TO PHYSICAL EXERCISES

- Dislike of physical activity—lack of enjoyment with it
- Lack of time
- Burden of excessive weight
- Depression
- Loneliness
- Lack of motivation
- Lack of support
- Cardiovascular, pulmonary, neurological, psychiatric, or orthopedic illnesses that limit the patient's capacity to exercise
- Discouragement and fears due to previous injuries
- Embarrassment to exercise in the presence of others
- Lack of access to an exercise facility
- Low self-confidence
- Negative attitude: "I'll never make it."
- Fear of having a heart attack or a cardiac arrest
- Difficulties in changing behavioral patterns
- Asthma
- Back problems
- Knee arthritis or torn ligament
- Foot pain due to heel spurs or stress fractures
- High blood pressure

BASIC RECOMMENDATIONS FOR AN EXERCISE PROGRAM

A. Prior to the beginning of the exercise program, the primary care physician or cardiologist recommends the time that should be daily spend doing the exercises (fifteen minutes, thirty minutes, etc.) and pace of gradual increments.
B. An orthopedic consultation is desirable to determine the kind of exercises that are allowed and those that should be avoided. This will prevent unnecessary injuries.
C. Nonweight-bearing and low-impact activities, such as simple walking, water exercises, chair exercises may be necessary in some cases.
D. Careful attention must be paid to the possibility of orthopedic injuries, behavioral reactions to exercise such as a development of antagonistic or distasteful attitude toward it, changes in blood glucose levels, such as hypoglycemic reaction, if the patient is on insulin or antidiabetes medications, exercise-induced severe hypertension or significant tachycardia (undue acceleration of the heart rate).
E. It is very important for you to select the type of exercises you like best since the program requires long-term adherence.
F. Goals must be set.
G. The start should be *slow and progressive.*
H. Keep track, record what you do. For example, how much you walked and at what speed. This will evaluate your progress, and you'll know what you've accomplished.
I. Sometimes—not always—you may consider doing workouts with a partner.
J. Do not have excuses to avoid your daily exercise. Rains and storms should not be an impediment. Do it at home. If you "don't have time," I suggest you do the best you can to find it! Your health is more important than . . . whatever!
K. If your business, profession, family, church activities demand more of your time, always remember that if obesity maims you or kills you, you'll have no business, no profession, no family, and no church activities.
L. Avoid getting bored with your program: alternate yoga with swimming, bicycling with stacking wood, and so forth.

ORTHOPEDIC COMPLICATIONS

Weight-bearing joints suffer from obesity. Some patients tolerate excessive weight better than others.

There is a popular belief that obesity greatly affects the lower back. Studies, however, proved a tenuous association at best. Acute low back pain affects most of the adult population at some point in their lives. An estimated 84 percent of the population in industrialized countries suffer from low back pain, and many of these individuals are not obese. Some studies noted that patients improved their low back pain by losing substantial amount of weight, and others could not document such improvement.

Knee and hip osteoarthritis, particularly the former, *are definitely affected by obesity*. Why the knees are more victimized by excessive weight than the hips is not entirely clear.

The process that leads to pain and incapacity is called osteoarthritis (OA). With or without obesity and more accelerated and precipitated by obesity, OA starts with injury to the cartilage and then injury to the bone underlying it. This is followed by deformities that lead to stretching of ligaments or even their rupture. The resulting pain causes disability. Insufficient use of the joint leads to muscle weakness.

Individuals with knee OA do not usually have pain in the morning on awakening but will feel the pain going up and downstairs, walking or getting up out of a chair.

Patients feel better or worse on alternating periods until the disease is advanced when the pain becomes less episodic and more persistent.

Obesity causes OA by afflicting weight-bearing joints and inducing cartilage breakdown and also by concentrations of metabolic products that are affected by adipose or fatty tissue.

Orthopedics found that total knee prosthesis (replacement) of a knee in the severely obese functions and lasts as well and as long as prosthesis implanted in nonobese persons. There are more reservations concerning hip replacement: long-term survival of these implants may be abbreviated.

A PERSONAL TRAINER (Just in case you can afford one)

The morbidly obese person must be particularly careful while implementing a program of physical exercises to avoid injuries.

1. The personal trainer should be certified in fitness and have experience dealing with obese persons.
2. If you want a personal trainer and do not know where to find one, ask for a recommendation by the Sports Medicine Division or Physical Rehabilitation Department of a major hospital.
3. A trainer should not include a person with severe obesity in a class with other individuals who have normal weights.
4. Even sharing a class or exercise session with other obese people has limitations since obese people have different kinds of joint or other medical problems. The role of the personal trainer is to *personalize* the treatment.
5. Sometimes, sharing a class with other persons may not be effective and may be counterproductive.
6. Make sure your electrolytes are OK, particularly levels of serum magnesium and potassium. These can be affected by diuretics, and when their blood levels are lower than normal, arrhythmias (heart rhythm irregularities) may occur.
7. There are useful techniques to prevent injuries in the morbidly obese, such as the medical ball—that protects the knees and back—and water exercises. The ball attenuates the impact of exercise on the body and helps posture and balance.
8. Pre-exercise stretching is most important.
9. Skin care with special creams must be paid attention to and is available to deal with cellulitis, ulcerations, perspiration, skin dryness.
10. The types of shoes to be used during exercise should be recommended by an orthopedic physician or a knowledgeable trainer.

I truly hope that you'll find some application for these suggestions, and that their implementation will give you an easier ride. Enjoy it!

CHAPTER 17

DIET PILLS AND THE NEED FOR THEIR CAREFUL SCRUTINY

If you can't solve a problem, at least, try not to make it worse than what it is.

Every time you are offered a weight-reducing pill and you're told that it works wonders, always take a hard look at the suggestion.

The fact of the matter is that drug treatment of obesity has created more problems than solutions. Historically, drugs to induce weight loss have been largely unsuccessful, often the cause of serious side effects, and occasionally, fatalities. Yet millions consume them.

People like quick solutions for their problems.

It isn't necessarily incorrect to think that way. Trouble is that reality prevails over good wishes and intentions.

Diet pills do not solve the obesity dilemma. No pill and, in fact, no medical or surgical treatment of obesity per se represents a solution for the morbidly obese patient. More than that is needed.

Even weight-loss surgery, for all its merits—which are many—is just a contribution to the overall treatment of this disorder, but a solution per se, let's say, you undergo gastric bypass and cure obesity for good, is nonexistent.

Bariatric surgery provides you a mechanical way to limit food intake and reduces caloric intake and absorption, but it will only succeed if you have the motivation, discipline, and persistence to adhere to drastic dietary changes and regular exercise on permanent basis. So that magic pill that obese patients and pharmaceutical corporations have been dreaming of, it's a fantasy. It hasn't been invented yet.

You may wonder how it is possible that mankind has successfully completed extremely complex space and interplanetary missions and other extraordinary scientific tasks and, still, couldn't come up with a little pill to cure obesity.

But that's the way it is!

And it isn't because scientists haven't tried hard enough. They have, but without the desired results. At times, it took millions of dollars to develop a drug to treat obesity and billions to compensate patients who took it. (Please see below.)

The first attempts to treat obesity with drugs date back to the end of the nineteenth century when thyroid hormone was first used. Since that time, most drugs used to treat obesity have caused far more problems than satisfaction.

You may think that the use of thyroid hormone to induce weight loss belongs to the history books. Not quite!

I've seen patients who took thyroid hormone pills to lose weight, and I was consulted because of severe palpitations. One of these was an obese nurse who took this drug and developed "a racing heart and shortness of breath." She had developed an arrhythmia with tachycardia of 185 beats per minute. She had to be immediately hospitalized.

I've also seen several female teenagers medicated with thyroid hormone for weight-losing purposes who lost their menstruation and became emotionally unstable, shaky, fearful, and apprehensive. It took quite a while for them to go back to normality.

DRUGS THAT CAUSE LOSS OF APPETITE

In modern times, amphetamines are used to treat obesity. These medications curve the appetite. Drugs that do that are called anorectic.

Amphetamines are considered addictive drugs although not all of them have the same degree of addictive power. This led to restrictions on their use by the United States Drug Enforcement Agency (DEA).

The above does not mean that these medications should never be used. Sometimes, when used wisely and in a limited way, they may induce some weight loss and have positive although limited effects in the patient's overall management of obesity.

It is clear though that one should use extreme caution before taking drugs for obesity, and when this is done, their administration must be carefully scrutinized and preferably followed up or supervised by a medical team that specializes in bariatric medicine.

There are other common conditions such as hypertension, diabetes, and high-cholesterol blood levels that are not cured by pills either. These conditions cannot be cured but can be controlled. You discontinue your pills to lower your cholesterol or your blood pressure, and it won't take long before abnormal numbers recur.

The Fen-Phen Story

Fen-phen refers to the use in combination of fenfluramine and phentermine. These are prescription medications that had been approved by the FDA for many years (fenfluramine in 1973, phentermine in 1959) as appetite suppressants for the short-term (few weeks) management of obesity. There was another derivative of fenfluramine, called dexfenfluramine (Redux) that was approved in 1996.

In the case of fen-phen and dexfen-phen, no studies were presented to the FDA to demonstrate either the effectiveness or safety of the drugs taken in combination. In the early and mid-1990s, physicians often used these combined medications for extended periods of time as part of weight-loss programs.

A Fateful Day

On July 8, 1997, the Mayo Clinic reported twenty-four patients who had developed heart-valve disease after taking fen-phen. Five of them required valve-replacement surgery.

The same day, the FDA issued a public health advisory that described the Mayo findings. These were reported in the August 28, 1997, issue of the *New England Journal of Medicine*, along with an FDA letter to the editor describing additional cases. FDA had received over one hundred reports of cases of heart-valve disease in patients taking only fenfluramine or dexfenfluramine. No cases of valvular heart disease were reported in patients taking phentermine alone.

On September 15, 1997, the Food and Drug Administration asked the manufacturers to voluntarily withdraw both Pondimin (fenfluramine) and Redux (dexfenfluramine) from the market.

On July 9, 1997, the first national lawsuit was filed alleging that the manufacturers of the diet drugs had failed to properly warn physicians and consumers concerning the dangers of these diet drugs.

On October 7, 1999, the manufacturer agreed to a class-action settlement valued at 4.75 billion dollars to pay for the claims of patients prescribed Pondimin and Redux. On August 28, 2000, a judge granted final approval for the settlement. *CNN* reported on Wednesday, 23 April 2003, the drugmaker Wyeth put aside 14.6 billion dollars to cover liability costs.

In one study involving 291 patients who had been treated by Pondimin, Redux, and usually in combination of one of these drugs with phentermine, abnormal echocardiograms revealed that 27 percent of the total group were found to have developed aortic valvular leakage, also called insufficiency or regurgitation; 8 percent were found to have developed mitral regurgitation, and 3 percent both.

The same drugs were also found to cause "primary pulmonary hypertension" (PPH), a very serious disease of the pulmonary arterial branches that constrict too much and dilate too little, thereby raising the pressure in the pulmonary arterial tree.

Before developing new drugs to treat primary pulmonary hypertension, the disease was rapidly fatal with nearly two-thirds of patients having only three years of life after the diagnosis. New therapies allow 65 percent of patients survive longer than five years.

DRUGS' MECHANISMS OF ACTION IN THE TREATMENT OF OBESITY

They act by

1. reducing food intake by decreasing appetite,
2. impairing intestinal digestion and absorption of fats and carbohydrates
3. strategies that could be developed affecting fat production (lipogenesis) and fat destruction (lipolysis),
4. increasing energy expenditure (currently not recommended).

We will focus our attention on *1 and 2 categories*.

1. DRUGS THAT REDUCE FOOD INTAKE BY DECREASING APPETITE (CALLED ANORECTICS).

There are two substances in the brain that influence appetite: norepinephrine (NE) and serotonin.

These act on the so-called *receptors*.

To decrease appetite, these *receptors*, which are contained in nerve cells called neurons, *must be activated*.

A. NE RECEPTORS are called alpha 1 and beta 2 adreno-receptors.
Their activation results from drugs that either release NE from receptors or block NE reuptake at the neuronal junction.

There are a number of drugs that have this kind of action. They are called sympathomimetic drugs. Some of them have been restricted by the FDA (United States Drug Enforcement Agency) because of their addictive potential, for example, phentermine.

Sibutramine (Meridia) is available in five milligrams, ten and fifteen milligrams pills. Ten milligrams per day, as a single daily dose, is the recommended starting level. Doses higher than fifteen milligrams are not recommended, and extreme caution should be used in patients with a history of coronary artery disease, congestive heart failure, cardiac arrhythmias, or stroke.

B. SEROTONIN RECEPTORS

There are seven families of serotonin receptors. One family (*5-HT2c*) regulates appetite. *Its activation decreases it.* Activation of a serotonin receptor means that serotonin released from the receptor site is not allowed to reenter it, and therefore, the *serotonin reuptake is blocked.*

This action decreases appetite.

Examples of drugs that block serotonin reuptake are fluoxetine, sertraline, or fenfluramine.

2. DRUG THAT REDUCES DIGESTION AND ABSORPTION OF FATS

Orlistat is a potent inhibitor of a pancreatic lipase, an enzyme that reduces the intestinal digestion of fat. Understandably, the drug has little effect on patients eating a low-fat diet.

The drug is not absorbed to any significant degree, so side effects are intestinal (increased frequency and a change in the character of the stools due to undigested fat). Fat-soluble vitamins are lost with this medication, but multivitamins supplements solve this problem.

3. DRUGS THAT INCREASE ENERGY EXPENDITURE

Ephedrine and caffeine: these drugs have been approved by the FDA for an indication other than obesity.

BE CAREFUL ABOUT WEIGHT-LOSING PILLS

Fen-phen has not been the only drug that caused serious medical problems.

The so-called herbal fen-phen is a product that does not contain fenfluramine, dexfenfluramine, or phentermine. Products called herbal fen-phen often contain a combination of ephedra (an ephedrine-containing herb) and caffeine.

Herbal supplements for weight loss are not properly regulated by the government, and many weight-loss supplements do not warn users about the potential health problems that could result from taking the drugs. Some of these may cause depression, anxiety, and heart problems.

The stimulant ephedra, the most commonly publicized and widely used weight-loss supplement, has been linked with illness and death. It has been estimated that over three billion servings of ephedra are consumed by Americans yearly.

The FDA recently alerted the public about Chinese weight-loss products, Chaso (Jianfei) Diet Capsules and Chaso Genpi, because they pose a potential public health risk. Some people in Japan who took this drug have become gravely ill and some have died after consuming these diet products.

The FDA has advised its import operations personnel to be on the alert for Chaso Diet Capsules and Chaso Genpi.

In 2001, FDA issued a nationwide alert on the recall of thirteen Treasure of the East herbal products because the products contain a toxic component aristolochic acid that causes kidney damage.

Obesity drugs are, at best, of transient value in assisting some people to achieve modest weight loss. This is gained right back after the drugs are discontinued.

Only two drugs are currently approved for long treatment of obesity. Sibutramine (Meridia), which is dangerous for patients with cardiovascular disease (see above), and Orlistat (Xenical) which produces 5-10 percent weight loss.

The available medications to treat obesity should be supervised by professionals who have experience and special knowledge in the field of bariatric medicine and who will integrate this kind of management with the overall psychological and medical therapeutic aspects of each individual patient.

CHAPTER 18

NUTRITION AND OBESITY
BAD HABITS DIE HARD

It is healthier to focus on the science of nutrition than on the art of eating.

Many influences have been blamed for the existence of obesity: genes, slow metabolism, the environment, physical inactivity, psychological-emotional dysfunctions, physical ailments, adverse socioeconomic conditions, poor food choices.

Every one of these factors affects each person differently. Human beings are different to begin with. And so are the various influences on their lives. These are often complex, and sometimes, it is difficult to identify the culprit.

Be that as it may, facts speak for themselves. In the United States, one in two adults is overweight, and one in three is obese.

The economic cost of obesity is prohibitive. Public health efforts have been made to prevent and treat obesity, and it hasn't been always clear whether the attention should be focused on genetic, environmental, psychological, or nutritional factors.

Without minimizing the importance of any of the multiple contributing factors, two of them are clearly decisive: consumption of the wrong foods and insufficient physical activity.

Both may result from defective education, income, or other social conditions. People with adequate income have more options and opportunity to select better food products. The same can be said about regular exercises. So it is not surprising to see that obesity in the United States is a prevalent disease of the poor and minorities.

The technological advances we enjoy have drastically reduced the pace of physical activities since machines and computers have replaced muscular efforts and ambulation.

People sit for too long, food choices are terrible, fast-food chains continue to intoxicate the population with the wrong sugars and fats, food corporations mislead the public, and many eat away from home. This leads to excessive consumption of unhealthy products.

OBESITY AND DIET

The main components of the diet are called macronutrients. These include carbohydrates, fats, and proteins.

There seems to be an influence of macronutrients on the brain chemistry among obese persons, an influence that is not apparent in lean individuals. It isn't clear as yet the role that each macronutrient plays in sending signals to the brain that promote excess weight gain.

There's no uniform agreement on the composition of diets and their contribution to obesity. There are different theories, and their promoters think they are correct, and everyone else is wrong.

What follows is a succinct view of some of the main nutritional programs aimed at the treatment of obesity.

Weight Gain and Carbohydrates

Some investigators believe that excessive consumption of starches and simple sugars leads to obesity, regardless of the total energy (calories) intake.

The suggested mechanism to produce obesity would be the increased production of insulin caused by carbohydrates, particularly those of low-fiber content. Excessive amount of insulin in the circulating blood is called hyperinsulinemia. This is responsible for an exaggerated storage of fat (adipose tissue).

Foods with high glycemic index (GI) contain simple sugars that are rapidly absorbed by the gastrointestinal tract. Their absorption leads to a series of hormonal and metabolic reactions that promote further food consumption among the obese. So in these cases, the selection of the wrong foods creates a vicious cycle and the perpetuation of obesity.

Foods that contain a high GI cause higher insulin levels than those foods that contain a low GI.

Foods that contain a low glycemic index (GI) produce lower postprandial (postmeals) blood glucose and lower insulin levels. This means that there will not be a tendency to accumulate fat in different tissues.

The glycemic index then plays an important role on the fate of carbohydrates and related insulin reactions. Its activity significantly influences obesity, diabetes, and cardiovascular disease.

Many researchers have recommended an increased consumption of carbohydrates but only those that are complex and contained in whole grain.

Weight Gain and Dietary Protein

Some investigators believe that obesity is the result of excessive protein consumption in early childhood. In the United States, high-protein diets tend to be rich in fat too (i.e., meat).

Weight Gain and Dietary Fat

A high-fat diet increases the likelihood of obesity, and a low-fat diet reduces the risk of obesity.

Fat has the highest energy density of all the macronutrients.

ENERGY DENSITY AND OBESITY

Energy density refers to the energy (or amount of calories) present in a given weight of food.

Macronutrients, such as carbohydrates and proteins, provide four kilocalories per gram. Fat provides nine kilocalories per gram. Alcohol, seven kilocalories per gram.

Fat, therefore, has the highest energy density.

Energy-restricted diet is the essential ingredient of any obesity therapy.

A reduction in intake of five hundred kilocalories per day below the body's requirement should lead to a loss of one pound per week.

Diets that contain one thousand calories a day or less carry some risks and should be medically supervised. Supplementation with multivitamins and minerals is important. Very low-calorie diets cause hair loss, increased tendency to gallbladder stone formation, menstrual disturbances, and hair loss.

Most health care practitioners refrain from the use of severely restrictive diets. The risks of side effects are significant.

High Carbohydrate, Low-Fat Diets

The American Heart Association and the United States Department of Agriculture have published guidelines recommending macronutrient intakes.

The stage 2 National Cholesterol Education Program diet derives only 25 percent of the energy from fat and 7 percent of its calories from saturated fat and less than two hundred milligrams of daily cholesterol consumption.

The National Heart, Lung, and Blood Institute recommended in May 2001, 25 to 30 percent of total calories to come from fat with less than 7 percent coming from saturated fats.

High-fiber foods induce greater satiety. Epidemiological studies support the view that there is a reduced incidence of high body weight among individuals who consume a high-fiber diet.

There is evidence to support the notion that fiber-rich diets containing nonstarchy vegetables, fruits, and whole grains may be effective in both the prevention and treatment of obesity.

The higher the diet fiber content, the lower the weight. It has also been suggested that a high-fiber diet protects against obesity and cardiovascular disease by lowering insulin levels.

The daily average consumption of fiber in the United States per person is fifteen grams per day. It is advisable to increase fiber consumption to at least thirty grams per day.

Low Carbohydrate, High-Protein Diets (Atkins)

Four to five decades ago, diets restricted in carbohydrates with unlimited intake of foods high in protein and fat were proposed for the treatment of obesity; and since then, many millions followed them. Part of the justification offered to adhere to these diets was the fact that sugar has a low satiety value.

Another point was the ketosis that resulted from this diet. Ketosis is the excessive production and accumulation of ketone bodies in the body, such as acetoacetic acid that result from this type of diet and reduce the appetite, thereby contributing to weight loss.

High-protein diets carry nutritional long-term risks. By limiting carbohydrates, micronutrients, phytochemicals, and plant sterols will be missing in the diet. Secondly, the effects of ketosis include rapid loss of water, dizziness, nausea, fatigue, and tendency to low blood pressure. There is also increased calcium mobilization from the bones.

The long-term use of saturated fats and cholesterol increases the risk of coronary artery disease and atherosclerotic involvement in other arterial territories.

This diet may indeed cause short-term weight loss, but the potential hazards we just described don't make it a palatable diet from the scientific standpoint.

Summary of Diets for Obesity

Diet Description Fat Carbs Protein Examples

	% kcal	% kcal	% kcal	
High fat, low carbs < 100 g/day	55-65	< 20	25-30	Atkins
High protein				
Moderate fat reduction				
High carbs, moderate protein	20-30	55-60	15-20	Weight Watchers

Very lot fat, very high carbs
Moderate protein   <10-19   > 65   10-20   Pritikin Program

  < = under
  = over

And now, please turn the page—if I didn't do enough to discourage you from doing so—and see the completion of our journey.

EPILOGUE

We spend our lives drawing conclusions. Before reaching conclusions, we think. Then we decide whether we should act or not on a particular decision.

The thinking-concluding-deciding-acting sequence characterizes human behavior. Morbidly obese patients must go through this mental process when they consider the weight-loss surgical option.

What's more difficult: think, conclude, decide, or act? Does it depend upon the individual?

There are people who think reasonably well but cannot reach a conclusion. Others reach a conclusion but find it difficult to decide on a course of action. There are those who decide what to do, but when the time to act is ripe, they just can't do it.

And of course, there's a peculiar breed of individuals who are able to act decisively without thinking. Some of the U.S. presidents, notably so in recent history, comfortably and effortlessly fall into this category.

Since I'm not a psychologist, I decided to pose this question to a world-renowned expert on that field, Prof. Dr. Arnold A. Lazarus.

American Psychology listed Professor Lazarus as one of the ten most influential psychotherapists in America.

I asked him, "Thinking, concluding, deciding, acting—which of these phases is considered the most difficult, at least, for most human beings?"

I had the great privilege of getting his answer. And here it is.

"Ed, it is, as you indicated, difficult to generalize because of considerable individual differences. Nevertheless, if we apply learning theory and clinical observation to the issue, the conclusion is that cogitation (thinking and concluding) is easier for most people than reaching a decision.

"Clinically, most patients seem willing and able to obsess, and they get a vortex of thinking and concluding and then rethinking and reaching different conclusions. Meanwhile, they do nothing to change the situation but keep going round and round in their head."

"*Behavioral Activation* is regarded as one of the most potent ingredients of change (that means acting and doing something to change the status quo). But most patients seem to resist making behavioral changes. It takes considerable clinical skill to persuade them to take reparative action." And there's another angle to a person's conclusions. In the particular case of the morbidly obese, in order to decide whether weight-loss surgery should be done or not, he/she *must resort to other people's experience*.

The reason for that is obvious: the affected person never had obesity surgery. Conversations with patients who underwent WLS, dialogues with health care practitioners with experience on the field, reading educational material are all helpful and necessary.

Having WLS is, indeed, a very important decision. Few operations can so drastically and permanently change the way a person looks, feels, thinks, works, eats, drinks, sits, stands up, plays, goes on vacation, practices sports, interacts with his or her sexual partner, children, siblings, relatives, friends, acquaintances, coworkers, and social contacts of all kinds.

So if you feel you have trouble to go through the sequence describe above—thinking, concluding, deciding—do not believe for a moment that your response is abnormal. It is not. In fact, it would be abnormal to decide for WLS without carefully evaluating the pros and cons.

The learning process about morbid obesity and what to do about it must be comprehensive and methodical. I've exposed many obesity-related issues and described the benefits and risks of weight-loss surgery. I hope this knowledge will help you to make your decision a bit easier.

I'd also like to think that the reading of my book did not give you the impression that I endorse obesity surgery every time I see a patient who weighs over one hundred pounds.

Not only I'd avoid obesity surgery if I could, but I'd do my best not to prescribe unnecessary medications or approve procedures or operations for *any medical condition unless they are absolutely necessary.*

The decision to have WLS—or not—is easier for the doctor than it is for the patient. After the first interview and examination of a morbidly obese patient, a health care practitioner familiar with this condition has a pretty good idea whether he or she qualifies for surgery.

As a patient, your own evaluation is more arduous and traumatic. There are concerns about the possibility of operative and postoperative complications and also the extraordinary physical and psychological changes that follow obesity surgery.

Do you have the necessary mental energy to go on with an entirely different lifestyle that will clearly have multiple advantages but will also modify the dynamics of personal relationships—sometimes favorably, sometimes unfavorably—and the quality and quantity of food items you've been attracted to for so long?

THE DECISION PROCESS

With respect to morbid obesity and WLS (weight-loss surgery), there are three possibilities:

* **You absolutely qualify for bariatric surgery.**
  You require WLS because the risks of serious disability or death due to the disease are considerably higher than the risks of WLS.
* **You absolutely do not qualify for bariatric surgery.**
  Physical or psychological reasons contraindicate the operation (chapter 5).
* **You do not qualify at one point but might qualify in the future.**

Example: You suffer from a severe OCD (obsessive-compulsive disorder), and this was responsible for a weight excess of two hundred pounds.

Without correction or significant improvement of the mental disorder, WLS will not succeed. Effective psychotherapy and psychotropic drugs may allow the surgeon to proceed.

If you feel you should have a consultation with another professional, do not hesitate to obtain it.

The decision to undergo WLS is unique and can't be compared with any other type of surgery. Those who have a face-lift or breast augmentation or another kind of cosmetic surgery certainly change. But these are all "segmental changes" that take place in one or several areas of the body.

Obesity surgery changes the whole person. You'll always recognize someone who corrected heavy eyelids, had nose or breast reduction, or liposuction in abdomen and thighs. But it will be difficult to recognize a person who has been treated with bariatric surgery. After losing one hundred, two hundred, three hundred pounds or more, people don't look the same.

And don't feel the same either! Now they are self-assured, have gone through various adjustments in their marriages or relationships, work with more energy, play sports, don't feel sorry for themselves, and have dramatically improved or corrected their diabetes, hypertension, heart failure, knee, hips, ankles, and low back pains, sleep apnea, and other respiratory difficulties. They are no longer victimized by people who used to, overtly or in a disguised manner, upset them with expressions of disdain and rejection.

In the end, the successful result of the morbidly obese treated by WLS is not only due to a well-done operation. This is, of course, essential. But that is only part of the entire picture. It is the patient's mental attitude, *your* attitude that will decide what kind of life you're going to have.

Whatever changes occur following the operation, these will depend not only on having a small stomach pouch, but what you'll do with it.

Weight-loss surgery is far more than an important physical event. It is a revolution of the mind and the spirit. It's one last frontier in the fight for your life and the struggle for survival, a renewal of hope, the liberation of long-contained and deeply rooted desires and aspirations, a commitment to secure a productive, healthier, and happier life, and be available at the right place and at the right time when those you deeply care about badly need you.

I hope all your dreams will come true!

Be well and take care of yourself.

My genuine best wishes.

APPENDIX 1

OBESITY AND SCUBA DIVING

Divers who are overweight (BMI greater than thirty kilograms/m_2) carry higher risks.

These are the reasons:

1. Decompression sickness
2. Cardiovascular disease (hypertension)
3. Diabetes (blood glucose fluctuations)
4. Impaired pulmonary function (hypoxia, CO_2 retention)
5. Deficient physical fitness
6. Decreased ability for self-rescue
7. Decreased buddy-rescue capacity
8. Higher risk of panic in stressful situations

Higher risks of decompression sickness have been noted in older divers. This may be due to the increased skin fold thickness (percentage body fat) and the increased incidence of cardiovascular disease commonly present in the obese.

When a person dives, nitrogen dissolves in all body tissues in proportion to the gas solubility and the blood flow to the tissue. "The bends" is the joint pain that expresses the nitrogen bubbles presence. The water content of the joints facilitates the gas solubility in those regions.

Nitrogen is also very soluble in fat. Because of that, nitrogen bubbles are produced in excess. If these bubbles find their way into the venous system, they travel to the lungs (pulmonary emboli). If the amount of bubbles is significant, they block the pulmonary artery branches and can cause severe shortness of breath and may be life threatening.

On occasions, bubbles that reach the right atrium via the venous system, instead of moving to the lungs through the right ventricle and the pulmonary artery, choose to pass from the right atrium to the left atrium through an opening called foramen ovale. From the left atrium, the bubbles go into the left ventricle, and from here may travel to the brain and cause a stroke.

It has been estimated that divers whose weight is more than 20 percent in excess should not be allowed to dive until they normalized it.

CHILDHOOD OBESITY
A GROWING AND
SERIOUS CONCERN

In the United States, 15 percent of children aged six to nineteen years and about 10 percent of preschoolers are overweight.

Rising incidence is seen in boys and girls and across all ages, racial groups, and geographic boundaries. This phenomenon is not only seen in the United States, but many other countries as well.

Risk factors involve genetic predisposition and environment. Families show heritability levels of 30 to 40 percent.

Childhood obesity is a risk factor for adult obesity.

Regrettably, many overweight children suffer obesity-related illnesses before they reach adulthood. Most overweight children between five and ten years of age suffer from hypertension or blood lipids abnormalities. Type 2 diabetes is common too. And in severe cases of childhood obesity, life-threatening conditions, such as obstructive sleep apnea, pose additional concerns.

Parental obesity is an important factor in many overweight children. So when treatment approaches are considered, the entire family must be counseled.

The impact of obesity in children is not only physical. Mood disorders and low self-esteem are common, the quality of life is affected, and there are negative social consequences.

Therapy strategies to deal with childhood obesity include behavior modification, techniques directed to reduce caloric intake and increase energy expenditure. Prolonged TV and video games exposure are particularly dangerous.

Diet programs must be carefully supervised. In the 1970s, there were reports of sudden death among adults using protein drinks. Dietary restrictions may also lead to hypokalemia (low blood levels of potassium), and dangerous arrhythmias may occur.

The treatment of obese children is as difficult as the treatment of the obese adult, if not more. Socioeconomic problems, parental obesity, addiction of kids to TV, and video games, as well as hamburgers, hot dogs, fries, cheesecake, chocolate, candy bars, and ice cream, so much part of our culture, make the conversion to an appropriate diet difficult.

In children, the management of obesity is particularly challenging. The professional in charge must be careful in balancing the caloric needs of the child without endangering his or her pace of growth or precipitating an eating disorder.

Frequent handicaps include inadequate training on how to counsel patients about weight loss and the poor reimbursement for obesity-related services.

Therapy success is based on the following:

- Establishing healthy dietary and physical activity behaviors early in childhood
- Family participation
- Public health policy

The main obstacles in approaching the therapeutic management of children's obesity are (a) insufficient awareness, and (b) the unwillingness to recognize the immensity of the problem.

Only those who realize how important and dangerous childhood obesity is will have a chance to deal with it effectively.

APPENDIX 3

LEPTIN AND GHRELIN

Leptin is a hormone that is produced by fat cells, called adipocytes.

It was discovered a decade ago, helps to regulate body weight, and continues under investigation.

Once leptin is released into the circulation, it works on an area of the brain called the hypothalamus (lateral and medial regions) by binding to leptin receptors and activating signals that regulate energy balance by reducing appetite and increasing energy expenditure through sympathetic system stimulation.

Absence of leptin produces massive obesity in mice and in humans. Treatment with leptin (experimental) decreases food intake in mouse and the leptin-deficient humans.

Most obese animals and persons have high blood levels of leptin. Since leptin acts by reducing appetite, it would be logical to think that an excess of leptin, circulating in a person's blood, would lead to weight loss.

So the offered explanation for the high levels of leptin in the obese is *leptin resistance*.

A clinical trial with leptin has been reported. In lean subjects treated for four weeks and in obese subjects treated for twenty-four weeks, a modest loss of weight was noted. The local irritation at the site of injection limits the use of this preparation. A long-acting leptin preparation might improve the use of this drug.

Ghrelin

This is a peptide (as leptin is) and recently received special attention because of its participation in the regulation of appetite. This hormone's synthesis occurs predominantly in epithelial cells lining the fundus of the stomach with smaller amounts produced in the placenta, kidney, pituitary, and hypothalamus.

At least, two major biologic activities have been ascribed to ghrelin:

- Stimulation of growth hormone secretion
- Regulation of energy balance: in both rodents and humans, ghrelin functions to increase hunger through its action on hypothalamic feeding centers. Ghrelin also appears to suppress fat utilization in adipose tissue.
- Blood concentrations of ghrelin are lowest shortly after consumption of a meal then rise during the fast just prior to the next meal.

Experimentally, the injection of ghrelin in the hypothalamus of rodents stimulated the animals' feeding and lead to weight gain.

Recent data suggest that short-term administration of ghrelin to humans stimulates appetite and food intake in humans. It seems to be potentially important in influencing appetite through action in the central nervous system.

The precise physiologic role of ghrelin, however, is under investigation.

There are other hormones and substances that influence appetite and food consumption: norepinephrine, insulin, steroids, dopamine, serotonin, acetylcholine, and others, but their discussion is beyond the scope of this book.

THE AMERICAN SOCIETY FOR METABOLIC AND BARIATRIC SURGERY (ASMBS), THE SURGICAL REVIEW CORPORATION (SRC), THE UNITED STATES CENTERS OF EXCELLENCE, AND THE OBESITY SURGEONS WHO BELONG TO THEM

When you look for good results in any human endeavor, choose nothing but the best.

The American Society for Metabolic and Bariatric Surgery is the largest society for this specialty in the world. The purpose of the society is to advance the art and science of bariatric surgery by continued encouragement of its members to

- pursue investigations in both the clinic and the laboratory;
- interchange ideas, information, and experience pertaining to bariatric surgery;
- promote guidelines for ethical patient selection and care;
- develop educational programs for physicians, paramedical persons, and lay people;
- promote outcome studies and quality assurance.

The leadership of the ASMBS recognized that there was a need to identify the centers, hospitals, and surgeons that reach levels of excellent performance. These ideas lead to the formation of the Surgical Review Corporation, which is an independent, nonprofit organization that took the responsibility of implementing the strict requirements that are necessary to be named as a Center of Excellence.

The objective of the SRC is not to limit bariatric surgery to a few, well-known centers. So many patients are in need of this treatment that the SRC wanted to identify the doctors who produce the best results. Poor results "are not acceptable."

The SRC has recently announced the launch of its new International Bariatric Surgery Center of Excellence Program in an effort "to establish consistent standards for bariatric surgery not only in the United States but throughout the world."

The selection is based upon physician-staff experience and credentials, incidence of surgical-related complications and mortality rates, appropriate equipment for management of morbidly obese patients, quality of postsurgical care, ongoing quality and improvements programs, and ability of patients to maintain their weight loss.

It takes a very good training, experience, skill, talent, hard work, and proven dedication to be selected as a surgeon in a Center of Excellence.

WEB SITES, RESOURCES, AND SOURCES OF ADDITIONAL INFORMATION

WEIGHT CONTROL

American Society for Metabolic and Bariatric Surgery
7328 West University Avenue, Suite F
Gainesville, FL 32607 (USA)
352-331-4900 (phone)
352-331-4975 (fax)
http://www.asmbs.org
E-mail: info@asmbs.org

American Society of Bariatric Physicians
303-770-2526
http://www.asbp.org

American Obesity Organization
www.obesity.org

International Bariatric Surgery Registry (IBSR) formerly known as the National Bariatric Surgery Registry (NBSR)

U.S. Centers for Disease Control and Prevention

U.S. Surgeon General

**U.S. Department of Health and Human Services
National Institutes of Health
Weight-Control Information Network**

1 Win Way
Bethesda, MD 20892-3665
202-828-1025 (phone)
202-828-1028 (fax)

Web site: http://www.win.niddk.nih.nih.gov
E-mail: WIN@info.niddk.nih.gov
Toll-free number: 1-877-946-4627

www.amedeo.com

www.asbs.org

www.foodanddiet.com

www.obesity-online.com

www.obesitysurgery-info.com

www.obesitysurgery.com

www.pulseamerica.org

ALCOHOL
1-800-ALCOHOL

This hotline is available twenty-four hours a day, seven days a week. Offers counseling and assistance in finding local treatment centers.

Alcoholics Anonymous Inc.
General Service Office
PO Box 459
Grand Central Station
New York, NY 10163
212-870-3400

CARDIOVASCULAR HEALTH
American Heart Association
National Center
7272 Greenview Avenue
Dallas, TX 75231-4596
800-242-8721

National Heart, Lung, and Blood Institute
Information Center
PO Box 30105
Bethesda, MD 20824-0105
301-251-1222

DIABETES
American Diabetes Association Inc.
1660 Duke Street
Alexandria, VA 22314
800-232-3472

National Diabetes Information Clearing House
One Information Way
Bethesda, MD 20892-3560
301-654-3327

DRUGS
National Institute on Drug Abuse
800-662-4357

Narcotics Anonymous
www.na.org

GENERAL HEALTH SERVICES AND INFORMATION

National Library of Medicine
8600 Rockville Pike

Bethesda, MD 20894
800-272-4787

MENTAL HEALTH ORGANIZATIONS

The National Mental Health Association
www.nmha.org

Mental Health Net-Self Help Source Book
mental health.net/selfhelp

NUTRITION

National Center for Nutrition and Dietetics (NCND)
216 West Jackson Boulevard, Suite 800
Chicago, IL 60606-6995
800-366-1655

National Cholesterol Education Program
NHLBI Information Center
PO Box 30105
Bethesda, MD 20824-0105
301-251-1222

SEXUAL DYSFUNCTION

Female Impotence
www.healthfind.org/health/female+impotence

Impotence Intitute of America
800-669-1603
www.impotenceworld.org

The Society for the Scientific Study of Sexuality
PO Box 416
Allentown, PA 18105-0416
Phone: 610-530-2483

www.SexScience.org

SMOKING

American Cancer Society
National Office
1599 Clifton Road NE
Atlanta, GA 30329
800-ACS-2345

American Lung Association
1740 Broadway, 14th Floor
New York, NY 10019-4374
800-586-4872

American Heart Association
National Center
7320 Greenville Avenue
Dallas, TX 75231
800-AHA-USAI

STROKE

National Institute of Neurological Disorders and Stroke
NINDS Information Service
Building 31, Room 8, A06
Bethesda, MD 20892

National Stroke Association
300 East Hampden Avenue, Suite 200
Englewood, CO 80110-2622
800-787-6537

American Stroke Association
888-478-7653

GLOSSARY

Abdominal angina. Abdominal discomfort caused by obstruction of an artery that supplies blood to the intestines.

Abdominoplasty. Also known as tummy tuck. It is a major cosmetic surgery that removes excess fat and skin from the abdominal area.

Ace-inhibitor (angiotensin-converting enzyme inhibitor). A drug used to treat hypertension and heart failure.

Adhesion. Scar tissue that unites two body parts that are not normally united, e.g, segments of intestines bound by scar tissue resulting from previous abdominal surgery.

Adipose. A fat tissue.

Adjustable gastric band (AGB). A silicone band placed by laparoscopy around the upper portion of the stomach, creating a small stomach pouch. It contains an apparatus on the inside like an inner tube that can be filled or emptied of water by using a port that is placed under the skin in the chest or side. Filling the tube with water results in a tighter constriction and slower emptying of the upper stomach pouch into the lower stomach.

Adrenaline. Also known as epinephrine. A hormone produced by the adrenal glands that increases the heart rate and relieves bronchial spasm.

Aerobic exercise. Exercise in which the muscles utilize oxygen (*aerobic* means "with oxygen." Examples are walking, running, swimming, skiing, cycling).

Anaerobic exercise. Exercise that is performed in short, intense bursts and does not utilize oxygen. For example, weight lifting.

Anastomosis. Surgical connection between two structures.

Aneurysm. Focal dilatation of an artery that results from weakness of the arterial wall.

Angina pectoris. Chest pain or discomfort due to deficient blood supply to the heart muscle.

Angiogram or angiography. X-ray picture of arteries that have been injected with a radio-opaque substance.

Angioplasty. Opening of a blocked artery by the use of a balloon.

Anorexia nervosa. A disease seen most frequently in young women characterized by intense fear of becoming obese. These patients have aversion to food and lose significant amount of weight. It is a serious disorder and it may be life threatening.

Anorexia. Poor appetite.

Anticoagulant. Blood thinner. Prevents blood clotting or delays it.

Antihypertensive. A drug use to lower high blood pressure.

Aorta. The largest artery in the body. It originates in the left ventricle of the heart and carries blood to the rest of the body.

Aortic valve. The valve between the aorta and the left ventricle.

Arrhythmia. Abnormal heartbeat: fast, slow, or irregular.

Arterial spasm. Constriction of an artery.

Arteriosclerosis. Hardening of the arteries.

Artery-arteries. Blood vessels that carry fresh, oxygenated blood throughout the body.

Artery. A blood vessel that carries oxygen-filled blood away from the heart to the organs and tissues.

Arthritis. Inflammation of a joint.

Ascending aorta. The first portion of the aorta takes off from the heart's left ventricle.

Asthma. A respiratory disease that causes bronchial spasms (constriction of the bronchial tubes) causing wheezing, coughing, chest tightness, and shortness of breath.

Asymptomatic. Without symptoms of disease.

Atherogenic. Any substance that contributes to the formation of atherosclerotic plaques.

Atheroma. Localized fatty material that forms a *plaque* inside the arteries and causes varying degrees of arterial obstruction.

Fatty deposit on the inner lining of an artery.

Atherosclerosis. A process of *atheroma* formation that primarily affects the inner layer of an artery and forms the atherosclerotic *plaque*. The reaction that involves other layers of the artery causes hardening of the vessel's wall that is called *arteriosclerosis*.

Buildup of atheromas that form the atherosclerotic plaques. These may or may not block the arteries significantly depending upon their size.

Atrial fibrillation. Irregular heartbeat produced by shivering of the atrial chambers.

Atrium. One of the two small upper chambers of the heart.

Bariatric. The field of medicine that deals with weight loss.

Bariatric surgery. Operations done in the stomach and sometimes the intestines too that result in weight loss. All weight-loss procedures restrict the size of the stomach. Some of them also prevent the absorption of calories and nutrients by bypassing a portion of the small intestine.

Bariatrician. Specialist in obesity.

Beta-blocker. Drug used to treat angina pectoris, hypertension, arrhythmias, heart failure, familial tremor, migraine headaches, and glaucoma.

Beta-carotene. An antioxidant found in orange and deep-yellow fruits and vegetables that converts into vitamin A in the body.

Bile. A greenish yellow fluid secreted by the liver that removes waste products and helps break down fats during digestion.

Biliopancreatic diversion (BPD). This is a classic malabsorptive procedure. It does not dramatically reduce the size of the stomach, and yet weight loss can be very significant. Since the size of the stomach is not dramatically reduced, patients can eat. However, the food bypasses the duodenum and all the jejunum and results in a number of serious malabsorption complications.

Binge eating disorder (BED). Episodes of binge eating that occur at least two days a week for a period of about six months. Patients describe loss of control and usually do it when they are alone. Food is consumed in large amounts over a period of about two hours.

Biopsy. A diagnostic test in which a small sample of tissue is removed from the body and examined under the microscopic. It helps to determine if a tumor is benign or malignant, but it is also useful to define other disorders.

Bipolar disorder. Also known as manic-depressive disorder. It is characterized by episodes of euphoria alternating with severe depression.

Blood clot. A clump of accumulated blood.

Blood pressure. Pressure or force exerted by the blood inside the arteries, resulting from the heart's pumping action.

Body mass index (BMI). Method of calculating degree of excess weight based on weight and body surface area.

BMI. *See* body mass index

Bradycardia. Slow heart rate (under sixty beats per minute). It may be normal or abnormal.

Bronchodilator. A medication that dilates constricted airways. It is used in asthma and some cases of chronic obstructive lung disease.

Bruit. Sound detected by the stethoscope that indicates some degree of arterial blockage by atherosclerotic plaques. Its detection is most useful to diagnose carotid artery disease.

Bulimia. An eating disorder. Binge eating followed by self-induced vomiting or laxative abuse.

Cancer association with obesity. Obesity is definitely associated with various cancers.

Cardiac. Pertaining to the heart.

Cardiac arrest. Cessation of the heartbeat.

Cardiac catheterization. A procedure that involves the insertion of a fine tube (catheter) into an artery, usually in the groin area, and passing the tube into the heart. It is done under local anesthesia. It evaluates the status of the heart function and valves, and it is usually used in conjunction with the *coronary angiogram*, which identifies obstruction of coronary arteries, their precise locations and severity. It is often an indispensable tool in the diagnosis and treatment of heart disease.

Cardiac output. The amount of blood the heart pumps through the circulatory system in one minute.

Cardiac Rehabilitation Program. A medically supervised exercise program attended by people with cardiac disease. Additional counseling is provided on diet, smoking cessation, stress control, and behavior modification.

Cardiac ultrasound. *See echocardiogrphy*

Cardiology. Study of the heart and its function in health and disease.

Cardiomyopathy. A disease of the heart muscle that often result in deterioration of the heart's pumping ability.

Cardiovascular risk factors. These are factors that increase the risk of cardiovascular disease. Examples are hypertension, diabetes, serum lipids abnormalities, sedentary lifestyle, smoking, family history, stress, poor eating habits, age (over forty-five in males and over fifty-five in females), elevated C-reactive protein, homocysteine lipoprotein (a) levels or being a postmenopausal female.

Cardiovascular system. Also known as the circulatory system. It consists of the heart and all the blood vessels (arteries and veins) that circulate blood throughout the body.

Cardioversion. Conversion of an abnormal cardiac rhythm to a normal one. It can be done with oral or intravenous medications or electricity by applying an electrical discharge in the patient's chest.

Carotid artery. A major artery located in the neck that supplies blood to the brain. (There are two carotid arteries, right and left.)

Carotid endarterectomy. A surgical procedure performed when the carotid arteries are blocked with atherosclerotic plaques.

Cellulitis. Bacterial infection of the skin involving the deeper subcutaneous layers. Edema of legs and venous insufficiency with skin damage and ulcerations so commonly seen in morbidly obese patients facilitates it.

Centers of Excellence. Institutions and surgeons selected by the American Society for Bariatric Surgery all over the United States that have shown consistent good results from bariatric surgery and have superior infrastructure organization.

Cerebral embolism. A blood clot that is carried by the bloodstream to the brain where it blocks an artery.

Cerebral hemorrhage. Bleeding within the brain resulting from a ruptured blood vessels due to hypertension, aneurysm, or head injury.

Cerebral thrombosis. Formation of a clot inside a cerebral artery.

Cerebrovascular accident. *See also* stroke

Cholesterol. One of many fatty substances that circulate in the blood stream and contribute to atherosclerosis. It is produced by many cells, mostly liver cells.

Chronic obstructive pulmonary disease (COPD). Obstruction and chronic inflammation of bronchial tubes (chronic bronchitis) or destruction of the respiratory units, alveoli (emphysema). The most frequent cause of COPD is smoking.

Comorbidity. The coexistence of two or more disease processes. Morbid obesity is associated with numerous comorbidities (chapter 1).

Conduction system. Electrical wiring system of the heart—also called bundles—that transmit electrical current that will stimulate the heart and cause its contraction.

Congestive heart failure. Weakened heart muscle resulting in fluid accumulation in lungs, liver, lower extremities, and other parts of the body.

COPD. *See* chronic obstructive pulmonary disease

Coronary arteries. Arteries that supply blood to the heart muscle.

Coronary artery disease. Narrowing of coronary arteries by atherosclerotic plaques.

Coronary bypass surgery. "Bridge" created by a segment of vein removed from the leg or arm that connects the aorta to a coronary artery below a severe coronary artery obstruction (*venous bypass graft*) or a thoracic artery called internal mammary artery (*internal mammary artery bypass graft*).

CPAP machine (*continued positive airway pressure machine***).** It is used to deliver oxygen to a sleeping person who suffers from sleep apnea.

CPR. *See* cardiopulmonary resuscitation

Cyanosis. Blueness of skin caused by insufficient oxygen in the blood.

DC shock. Electrical discharge applied to the patient's thorax to restore a normal rhythm.

Deep-vein thrombosis. A blood clot formed in a deep vein, usually in one of the lower extremities.

Defibrillator. A device that restores a normal heartbeat by delivering a brief electric shock to the heart muscle.

Depression. A mood disorder characterized by feelings of sadness, hopelessness, and helplessness combined with poor self-esteem, apathy, and withdrawal from social, personal, or family situations.

Dexfenfluramine (Redux). A weight-loss drug that was removed from the market in the late 1990s because it caused heart valves damage and also a potentially lethal disease called primary pulmonary hypertension.

Diabetes. A disorder in which the body is unable to use glucose properly.

Dialysis. A technique used for advanced renal failure that filters waste products.

Diastole. Each cardiac expansion and relaxation during which the heart chambers receive blood.

Diastolic blood pressure. When taking the blood pressure, this is the "bottom" one. It occurs when the heart relaxes in between heartbeats.

Digestive tract. Also known as the gastrointestinal tract. It consists of the mouth, throat, esophagus, stomach, small bowel, and large bowel.

Dilation. Process of enlarging a passage or anastomosis.

Dipyridamole stress test. It is a nuclear stress test. Dipyridamole is injected intravenously and causes a three to fourfold increase in coronary blood flow (more than exercise does). The injection of a nuclear substance too allows for detection of heart muscle areas that are blood-flow deficient.

Diverticula. A small pouch protruding through the intestinal wall frequently found in the colon but also esophagus and bladder.

Diverticulitis. Inflammation or infection of diverticula.

Diuretic. A drug that stimulates urine production. It is used to treat hypertension, heart failure, and edemas (fluid accumulation in lower extremities).

Dumping syndrome. Uncomfortable feeling of nausea, lightheadedness, upset stomach, diarrhea associated with the ingestion of sweets, high-calorie liquids, or dairy products following gastric bypass surgery.

Actually, this discomfort is beneficial to the patient because it discourages sweets consumption. This is believed to be part of the success of the Roux-en-Y procedure.

Duodenum. First twelve inch of small intestine immediately below the stomach. Bile and pancreatic fluids flow into the duodenum through ducts from the liver and pancreas.

DVT. *See* deep vein thrombosis

Dyslipidemia. Abnormal serum lipids levels—cholesterol, HDL, LDL, triglycerides, VLDL, or any of combination of the above.

Dyspnea. Shortness of breath.

Echocardiography. A painless procedure that uses sound waves to assess heart muscle and valve function.

Edema. Excessive fluid accumulation due to cardiac or extracardiac causes. It may be present in any parts of the body from the face down to the feet. When fluid accumulates in the lungs, it is called pulmonary edema.

Ejection fraction. The fraction (percentage) of blood ejected from the left ventricle with each cardiac beat. Normally it is 50 percent to 75 percent.

Electrocardiogram. A diagnostic procedure that records the electrical activity of the heart and serves to detect cardiac rhythm abnormalities, acute or past myocardial infarctions, and scars due to other cardiac disorders.

EKG. German abbreviation for electrocardiogram.

Embolus. A plug of material (such as blood clot, air bubbles, a tiny fragment of an atherosclerotic plaque, or miniscule fragment of a tumor) that can travel in the bloodstream and block an artery. The landing place of an embolus as well as its size determines the severity of the damage it causes (lungs, brain, spleen, legs, arms).

Esophagus. Tubelike structure that carries food from the mouth to the stomach.

Fatty liver disease. *See* nonalcoholic fatty liver disease

Fiber. The indigestible nutrient found in fruits and vegetables that passes through the digestive tract without being absorbed.

Gallstones: Gallbladder stones formed because the liver excretes too much cholesterol or the bile doesn't dissolve the excreted cholesterol.

Gastric bypass (GB). Operation designed to make nonfunctional a portion of the stomach.

Gastric reflux. *See* Gerd

Gastroesophageal reflux disease. Gastric juice moving up into the esophagus, causing inflammation of the esophagus mucosa and heartburn.

Gastrointestinal. Pertaining to stomach or intestines.

Gastroplasty. Operation for morbid obesity that reshapes the stomach.

Genetic. Pertains to transmitted hereditary characteristics.

GERD. *See* gastroesophageal reflux disease

Ghrelin. A hormone recently discovered that is secreted by endocrine cells within the stomach. Ghrelin blood levels increase prior to meals and in the face of food restriction or starvation.

Halitosis. Bad breath.

Heart attack. *See* myocardial infarction

Heartbeat. A contraction of the heart muscle that pumps blood into the arteries and reaches all organs and tissues of the body.

Heart conducting system. Bundles of the heart muscle that conduct electricity that stimulates the cardiac muscle and lead to its contraction.

Heart electrical system. *See* heart conducting system

Heart failure. *See* congestive heart failure

Herbal remedies. Natural substances that are not under the control of the FDA.

Hernia. Protrusion of a segment of bowel through the abdominal wall.

Hiatal hernia. A portion of the stomach that moved into the thorax.

High-density lipoproteins (HDL). Lipid fraction, good cholesterol; protects arteries.

Holter monitor. A portable device that records the electrical activity of the heart during a twenty-four-hour period.

Hormones. Chemicals, such as thyroid hormone or testosterone that are produced by the body and released directly into the blood stream to perform specific functions.

Hyperglycemia. Elevated blood glucose levels.

Hyperlipidemia. Increased blood lipids levels.

Hypotension. Low blood pressure.

Hypertension. High blood pressure. If prolonged and poorly treated, it leads to higher risk of strokes, heart failure, myocardial infarction, sexual dysfunction (erectile failure), renal failure, and diffuse arteriosclerosis.

Hypertriglyceridemia. High blood levels of triglycerides.

Hypotension. Low blood pressure.

Hypothalamus. A tiny although vital structure located at the base of the brain that regulates many body functions, including appetite and body temperature.

Hypoventilation. Impaired respiratory function leading to poor oxygen consumption.

Ileum. Ten feet of small intestine responsible for absorption. It extends from the jejunum to the cecum.

Implantable gastric stimulation system (IGSS). A pacemaker for the stomach. A small implantable battery pack is implanted under the skin and a wire extends to the vagus nerve of the stomach. It provides electrical stimulation to the nerve reducing appetite.

Infarction. Permanent damage done to a tissue or organ caused by a totally occluded artery, e.g., myocardial infarction, cerebral infarction.

Inferior vena cava. Collects blood from the lower part of body and carries it to the right atrium.

Inflammatory bowel disease. A term that refers to either of two chronic gastrointestinal disorders—ulcerative colitis or Crohn's disease.

Insulin. A hormone produced by the pancreas. It promotes the entry of sugar into the cells. It is essential for the body use of glucose as a source of energy.

Insulin resistance. Diminished ability of cells to respond to insulin in its action to transport glucose from the bloodstream into muscle cells.

Insurance policy exclusion. A denial of insurance coverage due to a specific exclusion, which sometimes excludes obesity surgery. This is considered the most difficult insurance denial to battle unless the insurance company failed to list this exclusion in its policy.

Ischemia. Deficient blood supply to any organ.

Ischemic heart disease. Heart disease that results from coronary atherosclerosis of coronary arteries and the deficient blood supply to the heart muscle that results from it.

Jejunum. Ten feet of small intestine responsible for digestion.

Kilogram. Measure of weight equal to 2.2 pounds.

Laparoscopy. Method of visualizing and treating intra-abdominal abnormalities with long fiber-optic instruments.

Large intestine. The portion of the digestive tract that extends from the small intestine to the anus. The sections of the large intestine include the cecum, ascending, transverse, and descending colon, sigmoid colon, and rectum.

Left anterior descending coronary artery. The largest coronary artery, which course down the front of the heart.

Left circumflex coronary artery. It flexes around the left side of the heart.

Left main coronary artery. Vital, initial portion of the coronary artery tree.

Left ventricle. The largest pumping chamber of the left side of the heart that ejects blood through the aorta into the circulation with each heartbeat.

Leptin. Hormone produced by fatty tissue that plays a role in appetite regulation.

Lipectomy. Surgical removal of fat tissue by cutting it off.

Liposuction. The process of removing excess of fat accumulated in pockets by a special suction device and using a small incision of one-fourth to two inches. It is the most common type of cosmetic surgery performed on men.

Low-density lipoproteins (LDL). Lipid fraction, bad cholesterol. Damages arteries.

Malabsorption. The body is unable to absorb nutrients of different kinas.

Malnutrition. A condition caused by a failure to eat or absorb the foods necessary to maintain adequate health.

Metabolic syndrome. This is a combination of obesity, insulin resistance, elevate plasma fatty acid levels, borderline or established diabetes, hypertension, and serum lipids abnormalities (syndrome X). It predisposes to atherosclerotic cardiovascular disease.

Morbidity. Pertaining to disease.

Morbid obesity. Body mass index (BMI) or forty or more.

Mortality. Pertaining to death.

Myocardial infarction. Permanent damage of the heart muscle that results from acute critical blockage of a coronary artery.

NIH. National Institutes of Health

Non-invasive procedure. Any diagnostic or treatment procedure in which no instrument enters the body.

Norepinephrine. Also called noradrenaline. A hormone that helps regulate heart rate and blood pressure by increasing heart rate and narrowing the blood vessels when the blood pressure drops below the normal level.

Obesity. Excessive weight due to excessive accumulation of fatty tissue.

Pancreas. An organ that lies behind the stomach that secretes enzymes and hormones, including insulin.

PET or PET scan. *See* positron emission tomography

Pituitary gland. A little gland indispensable to sustain life located at the base of the brain that produces hormones and regulates and controls other hormone producing lands and numerous body processes.

Plaque. A formation of cholesterol deposits inside arteries that may break and cause a clot formation or may progress in size and block the vessel.

Pulmonary emboli. Blood clots that reach the lungs, usually released from the lower extremities.

Pylorus. A muscular valve at the lower end of the stomach that controls the passage food into the duodenum.

Rectum. Final section of the large intestine that approximately measures nine inches long.

Restrictive surgery. A type of weight-loss procedure in which the size of the stomach is dramatically reduced.

Risk factors. *See* cardiovascular risk factors

Roux-en-Y gastric bypass. This procedure was named after César Roux, a Swiss surgeon. It creates a small stomach pouch, which is stapled horizontally separating it from the rest of the stomach. The small intestine is cut near the origin of the jejunum (second part of the small bowel), and the long portion of the jejunum is attached to the newly created small stomach. So food travels directly from the small stomach into the jejunum.

Since food is in contact with the digestive juices for less than the normal period of time, some malabsorption occurs.

Currently, this is the generally considered the best and safest bariatric procedure.

Saturated fats. Fatty acids whose carbon molecules are fully occupied by hydrogen atoms. Otherwise, they are called unsaturated. Saturated fats and found in meat and dairy products and can raise the level of cholesterol in the blood and increase the risk of coronary artery disease, disease of many other arterial territories, and certain forms of cancer.

Sepsis. Profuse number of bacterias in the bloodstream.

Sibutramin (meridia). A weight-loss medication.

Silent ischemia. Coronary heart disease that reduces blood supply to the heart muscle and yet is not expressed by symptoms of any kind.

Sleep apnea (obstructive sleep apnea). Frequent disorder in morbidly obese patients. It's an upper airway obstruction. Patients have disturbed sleep snore during the night and have daytime somnolence.

Sleeve gastrectomy: A surgical vertical resection of part of the stomach to restrict food consumption.

Spleen. An abdominal organ that contributes to fight infections in the body. It may be injured during weight-loss surgery.

Stomach pouch. Small receptacle left after stomach resection during weight-loss surgery. Usually holds three to nine ounces of food.

Stroke. Also known as cerebrovascular accident. Sudden damage to the part of the brain caused by an interruption in blood flow. It may result from a clot that travels from the heart chambers, aorta, or carotid arteries broken particles from atherosclerotic plaques, blockage of the carotid artery, blockage of a cerebral artery due to a plaque, or ruptured cerebral artery (cerebral bleeding).

Super morbid obesity. Two hundred or more pounds of weight excess or having a BMI of fifty or more.

Stress test. Test done for detection of coronary artery disease or to evaluate the patient's tolerance to exercise.

Syndrome X. *See* metabolic syndrome

Syncope. Acute, sudden loss of consciousness.

Systolic blood pressure. The highest of the two blood pressure numbers.

Tachycardia. Faster than normal heartbeat (normal heart rate sixty to one hundred).

Tachypnea. Faster respirations.

Thermogenic. Any food, drug, or activity that boosts metabolism.

Thrombosis. Clot formation inside an artery or a vein.

Thrombolysis. The breaking of a blood clot.

Thrombophlebitis. *See also* DVT (deep venous thrombophlebitis)

Thrombus: A blood clot that may form inside a cardiac chamber, an artery, or a vein

Thyrotoxicosis factitia. Clinical picture of hyperthyroidism provoked by inappropriate or excessive administration of thyroid hormone usually done for weight reduction purposes. It may cause serious problems including an arrhythmia called rapid atrial fibrillation.

Transient ischemic attacks (TIA). Temporary deficiency of blood supply to the brain that causes reversible neurological deficits in minutes or a few hours without causing permanent neurological damage (speech slurring, confusion and disorientation, visual deficits, weakness of an arm and leg).

Triglycerides. A group of fat lipids associated with cardiovascular disease when their blood levels are elevated.

Ultrasound. High-frequency sound vibrations, not audible to the human ear, used in medical diagnosis by producing an image or photograph of an organ or tissue within the body.

Unsaturated fats. Fatty acids whose molecules are not fully occupied by hydrogen atoms ions.

Upper Airway Obstruction. *See* sleep apnea

Valvular insufficiency. *See* regurgitation

Varicosities. Prominent, diseased veins, resulting from contractile deficiencies by the venous wall that lead to slow venous blood circulation, increased venous pressure and dilation of veins.

Vasoconstriction. Constriction of a vein or an artery.

Vasodilation. Dilation of a vein or an artery.

Venous insufficiency. Inability of the lower extremities veins to move the blood toward the heart, causing sluggishness of the venous circulation and formation of varicose veins.

Ventricular fibrillation. Chaotic, disorganized cardiac muscle contractions that is fatal unless quickly corrected.

Ventricular tachycardia. Abnormal rapid beating that originates in an excited, intrusive area of the ventricle that normally the ventricle does not produce.

Vertical banded gastroplasty. It is a purely restrictive weight-loss procedure. The stomach is stapled close to where the esophagus meets the stomach. The staples are placed vertically. This results in a very small stomach pouch.

Very low density Lipoproteins (VLDL). A type of lipid that increases the risk of coronary and vascular disease.

Vitamin B12. A vitamin found in food and supplements. It is absorbed in the stomach. Deficiency causes a condition called pernicious anemia.

VLDL. *See* very low density lipoproteins

Weight-loss surgery. *See* Bariatric Surgery

Yo-yo dieting. Losing and regaining weight multiple times.

INDEX

blood pressure. *See* hypertension
blood volume, 49-50, 53
Blount's disease, 36, 41
BMI. *See* body mass index
body mass index, 21, 25, 27, 32-33,
     37, 62, 84, 113, 115, 147, 173,
     196, 224
BPD/DS. *See* biliopancreatic
     diversion with duodenal switch
BS. *See* bariatric surgery
bulimia, 86
bypass
  gastric, 89-90, 97, 100, 103, 109,
     111-12, 125, 130-32, 136, 139-
     41, 156, 159
  small bowel, 131

C

calcium, 60, 100, 110, 132
calories, 15, 23, 26, 28, 90, 109, 111,
     168, 170, 187-89, 211
  spent with exercises, 168
cancer, 19, 34, 37-38, 82, 86, 107,
     116, 150, 152, 156, 223
  breast, 38
  cervical, 38
  colon-rectal, 38, 150
  endometrial, 34, 38
  esophageal, 38, 116
  prostate, 38
  renal, 34, 38
  uterine, 38
carbohydrates, 15, 22, 101, 183,
     187-88, 190
carbon dioxide retention, 77-78,
     196
cardiac, 32-33, 46, 48, 50, 53-55,
     57-59, 62, 75-76, 79, 82, 86,
     107, 109, 116-17, 155, 175,
     183, 196, 213-14, 216, 218,
     224-25
  abnormalities, 48

arrest, 32, 58, 79, 175
arrhythmia, 82, 183
cells, 54-55
chambers, 46, 50, 53, 75, 224
disease, 213
dysfunction, 58
muscle, 116, 218
output, 50, 213
rhythm disturbances, 116
standstill, 59
valves, 46
cardiomyopathy, 35
cardiopulmonary resuscitation, 59
cardiovascular disease, 19, 35, 40-
     41, 62, 113, 115, 170, 185, 188-
     89, 196, 205, 213, 225
  hypertensive, 48, 62, 75
carpal-tunnel syndrome, 36
Carrasquilla, Carlos, 122-34, 137-
     38, 154
cataracts, 34, 40
cellulitis, 40, 178
cerebral
  artery, 35, 65-66, 224
  hemorrhage, 35, 66-67
  infarction, 65
cerebrovascular disease, 64
Chapunoff, Eduardo, 4, 7, 17, 163
CHF. *See* congestive heart failure
childhood obesity, 6, 25, 60, 161,
     188, 198-99
children, 22, 28, 41, 134, 173, 193,
     198-99
China, 28
  obesity trend in, 28
cholesterol, 19, 23, 27, 33-34, 36,
     62, 112, 116, 181, 189-90, 207,
     217, 219, 223
chronic obstructive pulmonary
     disease, 82
circulatory overload, 49
circulatory system, 43, 49, 53, 57,
     74, 213-14

THE AUTHOR

Eduardo Chapunoff, M.D., is a diplomate of the American Board of Internal Medicine and the American Board of Cardiovascular Disease, a fellow of the American College of Physicians and the American College of Cardiology. He was a clinical associate professor of medicine at the University of Miami from 1985 to 1997.

He was the Medical Director of a St. Francis Hospital Institute, Miami Beach, and the acting chief of staff at the Veterans Administration Outpatient Clinic, Oakland Park, Florida.

Dr. Chapunoff has been included in the biographical records of Marquis Who's Who Publication Board, Personalities of America, Community Leaders of America (American Biographical Institute), and the International Who's Who of Intellectuals (International Biographical Centre, Cambridge, England). He was named International Man of the Year 1991-1992 (International Biographical Center, Cambridge, England).

He's the author of *Sex and the Cardiac Patient* **(1991)** and its Spanish version *El Sexo y el Paciente Cardiaco* **(1992),** which was also published in Argentina by Editorial Lidiun (1993). El Ateneo, one of the most prestigious publishing houses in South America, was its exclusive distributor. The English version sold in countries as distant as Singapore and Australia.

In 2004 he published *Answering Your Questions about Heart Disease and Sex*. This work was designated as the **Editor's Choice** by iUniverse Publishing and was a *finalist* for **ForeWord Magazine's 2004 Book of the Year Awards**. In October 2007 the book was published by **Hatherleigh, New York (distributor: Random House).**

Morbid Obesity and the Struggle for Survival was published in 2007 (iUniverse). *Morbid Obesity: Will You Allow it to Kill You?* is a revised and updated version of the former.

His latest work ***How Not to Drop Dead! A Guide for the Prevention of 201 Causes of Sudden or Rapid Death is currently in print (Xlibris)***

The author is completing the translation of all of his books into Spanish. These are expected to become available to the public in the first half of 2010.

The Customer's Research Council of America-2009- selected him as one of America's Top Cardiologists".

Dr. Chapunoff is currently the chief of cardiology at the Doctor's Medical Center and its six medical facilities, Miami, Florida.

His extracurricular activities include violin playing and oil planting. His artwork has been displayed in art galleries a number of times.

Visit his website: *www.dreduardochapunoff.com*